Atlas of Comparative Diagnostic and Experimental Hematology

Atlas of Comparative Diagnostic and Experimental Hematology

Second Edition

Clifford Smith and Alfred Jarecki

Foreword by Harold Tvedten

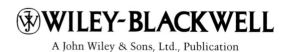

A John Wiley & Sons, Ltd., Publication

Library of Congress Cataloging-in-Publication Data
Smith, Clifford, 1952–
    Atlas of comparative diagnostic and experimental hematology / Clifford Smith and Alfred Jarecki; foreword by Harold Tvedten. – 2nd ed.
        p. ; cm.
    Rev. ed. of: A Color atlas of comparative diagnostic and experimental hematology / C.A. Smith . . . [et al.]. Wolfe, 1994.
    Includes bibliographical references and index.
    ISBN 978-1-4051-7107-6 (hardback : alk. paper)   1. Veterinary hematology–Atlases.   I. Jarecki, Alfred.   II. Color atlas of comparative diagnostic and experimental hematology.   III. Title.
    [DNLM: 1. Hematology–Atlases.   2. Mammals–Atlases. WH 17]
    SF769.5.S65 2011
    636.089′615–dc22

                      2011007528

A catalogue record for this book is available from the British Library.

This book is published in the following electronic formats: ePDF 9781444341713; ePub 9781444341720; Mobi 9781444341737

Set in 11/13 pt Minion by Toppan Best-set Premedia Limited, Hong Kong

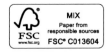

Contents

Foreword

I have been asked to write a foreword to the second edition of *Atlas of Comparative Diagnostic and Experimental Hematology*. It is an advantage to see the usefulness of this book from a different perspective than the editors and authors who work primarily with groups of animals in research settings. My background is in diagnostic laboratory medicine, including hematology, of mainly individuals of the common domestic animals, dogs, cats and horses in university and private veterinary hospitals. University and private veterinary hospitals sporadically work with samples from uncommon patients such as "pocket pets" including rats, guinea pigs and hamsters, monkeys, snakes, lizards, birds and fish. These plus other uncommon patients such as llamas, goats, sheep, marine mammals, etc., create a special challenge in one's laboratory. Good references are essential for proper hematological testing of the species being presented to us.

I have been mainly associated with the American Society for Veterinary Clinical Pathology, American College of Veterinary Pathologists and European Society of Veterinary Clinical Pathology through the years. More recently I have interacted with the Association for Comparative Clinical Pathology (ACCP), though I have interacted with laboratory professionals in toxicology and drug development over the last 35 years. I have been impressed with the quality of presentations at ACCP meetings aimed at improving the precision, accuracy and quality of laboratory testing by hematologists in toxicology and drug development in industry. I am also impressed with the quality, scope and value of the second edition of this book in this branch of hematology. I look forward to seeing it in print.

A book is a vital tool to aid people in performing their tasks. *Atlas of Comparative Diagnostic and Experimental Hematology* was written by professionals experienced in performing hematology testing in the toxicology and drug development environment. They are best qualified to describe well the current standard of laboratory practice in the field. The quality of this book reflects the time and effort taken to obtain, organise and present the appropriate information needed for us in the laboratory. Hematology is a visual, morphologic field and therefore an atlas is vital to answer questions that arise commonly by those working in the laboratory. Specialised atlases for each branch of hematology are needed. This second edition fills that role for testing of the comparative species and should be in each laboratory performing hematology testing on these animals. Considering the cost of laboratory testing and the investment in development of laboratory professionals to perform those tests well, the cost of a book is a very minor investment in producing correct and consistent results.

In addition to photographs in this atlas, which are required for proper classification of blood cells of these animals, there is abundant information on sample collection, artifacts and methodology, and descriptions of variations in hematology results due to factors such as species, breed, sex and age of the animals being studied. This information is of important and practical use for experimental design, sample collection, performing basic methods such as making blood or bone marrow smears, to performing more advanced methods such as flow cytometry and interpreting results in light of biological variation, pre-analytical errors in sample handling, method imprecision and therefore proper identification of a potential effect of a test compound. I complement the authors of the second edition and the drive and foresight of those others that encouraged and aided in its production. Production of this effective tool will have important and lasting effects on the quality of morphological evaluation in comparative diagnostic and experimental hematology.

Harold Tvedten DVM PhD, Dipl ACVP
Professor Emeritus, Department of Pathology
Michigan State University, East Lansing, Michigan

Introduction

Since the publication of the original *Color Atlas of Comparative Diagnostic and Experimental Hematology*, the Association for Comparative Haematology (ACH) has merged with the Animal Clinical Chemistry Association (ACCA) to form the Association for Comparative Clinical Pathology (ACCP). This second edition of the Atlas has again been enthusiastically encouraged and supported by members of this group. In more recent years, this group has forged many associations with wider groups such as the European Society of Veterinary Clinical Pathology (ESVCP) and the Association of European Comparative Clinical Pathology (AECCP).

The reasons for production of the original volume still exist – a limited number of related publications, variations in blood collection methodologies, inherent difficulties in methodology, etc. Since then, the discrepant data referred to in that edition have been more complicated due to an increased variety of analysers and analytical methods, although a better understanding of these factors has led to deeper understanding of the data produced and enabled enhanced interpretation of the results.

The design of toxicity studies is now well established and has been, and continues to be, refined such that the data are much better understood and can be interpreted in great depth. The increased number of people interested in comparative, diagnostic and veterinary hematology, reflected in the higher levels of qualification and number of interested groups, have made this publication even more relevant to today's environment.

Results obtained on any individual or group of individuals are dependent on an enormous variety of factors including pre-analytical factors such as species, strain, age, sex, diet, bleed site, nutritional status, husbandry procedures, stress levels (anxiety in particular will lead to splenic contraction, resulting in increased total white cell, differential and platelet counts), pregnancy, anticoagulant requirements, centrifugation speeds, storage temperature and so on; and analytical variability such as methodology, reagent quality, analyte stability, biological variability, artifacts, etc. Trying to assess what is normal for any particular assay or test, and whether there is an effect of pharmacological treatment, must therefore include an assessment of all of these factors, and be taken into account when comparing or interpreting data whether in a diagnostic situation or assessing treatment-related or toxicological effects. Due to inconsistencies in counting methodologies, reference ranges/normal ranges/typical values should be treated as guides and results more related to each other and indices than distinct ranges. Comparison with concurrent control groups in toxicological interpretation is critical for this environment.

Typical age-related ranges generated in our own laboratories are presented graphically with two standard deviations (95% confidence limits) from the mean for those species for which we have data.

Many publications have examined and described these relevant factors and so will not be further mentioned here except where the effects demonstrate abnormal or unusual blood and bone marrow cell morphology, or where these effects can lead to misleading data interpretation.

Many of the newer techniques developed in recent years have utilised the principal of flow cytometry, and the recent growth in interest in immunotoxicology to which this methodology is eminently suited, has stimulated rapid growth in this area. Therefore, in this edition the authors felt that the inclusion of some information on this technique and its applicability to comparative hematology would make a valuable and critical contribution.

Dedication

The untimely departures of our good friends Derek Hall, Mike Andrews and more recently Geoff Brown and Chas Mifsud, in conjunction with the retirement of John Collard, and Andy Walker leaving the industry, has delayed the production of a second edition. However, this project, kick started by Geoff and Chas (both valued friends and enthusiastic supporters), re-ignited the process and led directly to the publication of this work.

We would like to take this opportunity to thank all involved (past and present), our colleagues and employers (Covance and Sanofi-Aventis), contributors from both sides of "the pond" (and, indeed, the planet), and especially with thanks to our long-suffering families, for all their support and encouragement. There are too many members of the ACCP to mention individually, but to all members we extend our gratitude.

We truly hope that you, the reader, enjoy this work and that it proves to be useful in the course of your work.

In memory of Derek, Mike, Geoff, and Chas, and with special thanks to our wives, we dedicate this work.

Acknowledgments

The authors would like to acknowledge the contributions made by the following:

Mike Andrews (ex-GlaxoSmithKline UK Limited)
John Bleby (Sysmex UK)
Lisa Hulme-Moir (University of Glasgow, UK)
Lyn Lloyd (West Bar Veterinary Hospital, UK)
Anne Mathers (AstraZeneca UK Limited)
Wayne Melrose (University of Glasgow, UK)
Anne Pietersma (Astra Zeneca UK Limited)
Ian Roman (GlaxoSmithKline UK Limited)

We would especially like to thank Geoff Brown and family for contributing the chapter on bone marrow analysis, and Chas Mifsud for all the help and support provided early in this project. In addition, the chapter on flow cytometry supplied by Alaa Saad (AstraZeneca, Sweden) has made an enormous contribution to modern comparative diagnostic and experimental hematology by relating visual (microscopic) observations to the modern technologies now used in routine laboratories.

Many thanks are extended to the many members of the ACCP (too numerous to name individually) for their encouragement, but especially to the members of the ACCP committee for their help and support throughout the time taken to bring this project to completion.

It is of prime importance for us to also thank our employers (Covance Laboratories UK Limited) and also Sanofi-Aventis for their support in providing the means for us to be able to collect and discuss the material for this publication. Reference range data were provided by Covance Laboratories UK Limited with the exception of data for marmosets which were provided by Covance Laboratories Muenster. In addition, we must thank our colleagues who have had to take care of the fort during our meetings.

Lastly, we would like to record our thanks to our long-suffering families for all the hours spent in solitude (theirs and ours!), at a microscope and camera, in front of a PC, travelling to and from meetings, and numerous others tasks concerned with compiling a work such as this.

Thank you all.

1

Rodents

MOUSE

Introduction

Many strains of mouse (*Mus musculus*) are kept as pets, used in research and employed in preclinical studies. It is important to realise that not all hematological values may have stabilised before selection for toxicity studies, on average at around 10 weeks of age.

The descriptions detailed here are based on our experiences with CD1 mice, but most comments are equally applicable to most other strains.

Blood picture

Due to the high metabolic rate of mice red cells[1], erythrocyte counts tend to be high in comparison to those of larger mammals, typically in the range 7.0–11.0 × 10⁶ cells/μL. Hemoglobin values fall rapidly in young animals of both sexes as they mature, reflected in the mean cell hemoglobin concentration (MCHC), and are consistent with those of other mammalian species, i.e. in the range of 12.0–17.0 g/dL.

After birth mean corpuscular volume (MCV) values decrease rapidly in the first week, becoming fairly consistent between the sexes and stable across time by approximately 3 weeks of age. MCV and mean corpuscular hemoglobin (MCH) values reflect the small size of red cells in this species whilst the MCHC in mice tends to be close to 31.0 g/dL in fresh samples from mature animals.

Red cell distribution width (RDW) and hemoglobin distribution width (HDW) reflect the variability of the population of red cells, normal values tending to be similar to human with RDW in male animals slightly increasing with age whilst HDW reduces in both sexes.

As in humans, reticulocytes increase the erythrocyte count to normal adult levels after which they reduce to normal adult levels (around <5%), remaining stable throughout life.

Anisocytosis and polychromasia are prominent, although erythrocytes are not as susceptible to blood sample age/time-related shape changes as those of rats and do not show these effects to as great a degree.

Typical values for total white cell counts vary between different strains of mice but typically increase with age (more evident in male than female animals), and a diurnal variation may be seen[2].

Lymphocytes constitute the majority white cell population, rising with age and accounting for this effect in total white cell count; they are seen as a relatively homogeneous population in healthy subjects.

Neutrophil absolute counts are quite variable.

Monocytes are normally present in low numbers in peripheral blood in healthy animals, and usually contain vacuoles.

Eosinophils are normally present in low numbers in peripheral blood in healthy animals, although on occasion they may be increased with no obvious clinical or pathological cause. Basophils are rare in the peripheral blood of normal healthy individuals but may be increased following "milking" of the tail due to tissue basophils being expressed.

Large unstained cells (LUCs) constitute up to 5% of the normal population of circulating white cells, and reflect the same situation as in other species; increases are due to reactive, activated or atypical lymphocytes, or mononuclear cells.

Platelet counts are extremely variable[3,4,5], and platelets have smaller individual volumes than human platelets, typical values for CD1 mice being 4.5–11.6 fL. Platelet counts, volume estimations and population

Atlas of Comparative Diagnostic and Experimental Hematology, Second Edition. Clifford Smith, Alfred Jarecki.

statistics may be compromised by degranulation and clumping of platelets, and/or partial clotting of the sample; platelet count validity must be considered very carefully in the light of microscopic examination of the blood smear.

Typical ranges (Siemens Advia 120)

Due to the low numbers of monocytes, eosinophils, basophils and LUCs present in peripheral blood, this data is not expressed here.

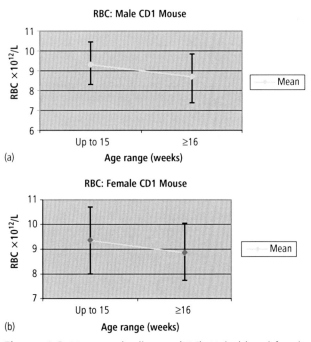

Figure 1.1 Mouse: hemoglobin (Hb). Male (a) and female (b) animals.

Figure 1.2 Mouse: red cell count (RBC). Male (a) and female (b) animals.

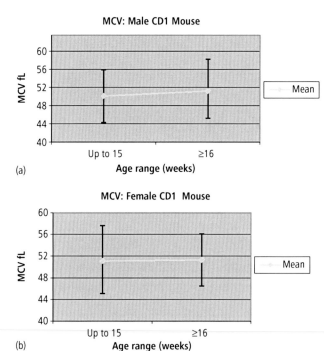

Figure 1.3 Mouse: mean cell volume (MCV). Male (a) and female (b) animals.

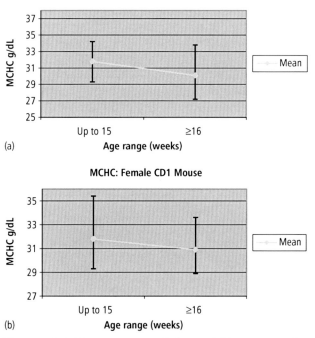

Figure 1.4 Mouse: mean cell haemoglobin concentration (MCHC). Male (a) and female (b) animals.

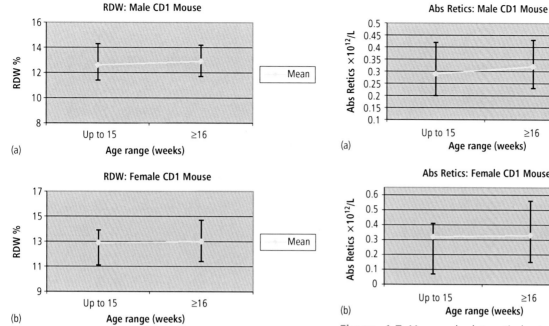

Figure 1.5 Mouse: red cell distribution width (RDW). Male (a) and female (b) animals.

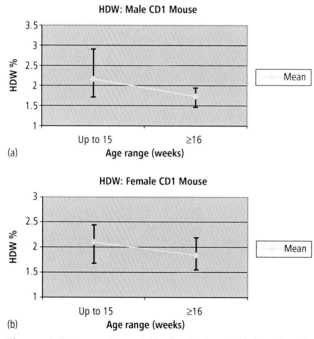

Figure 1.6 Mouse: hemoglobin distribution width (HDW). Male (a) and female (b) animals.

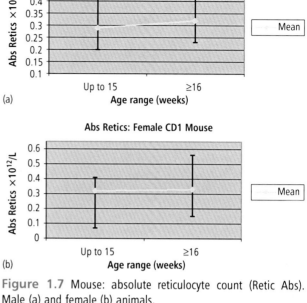

Figure 1.7 Mouse: absolute reticulocyte count (Retic Abs). Male (a) and female (b) animals.

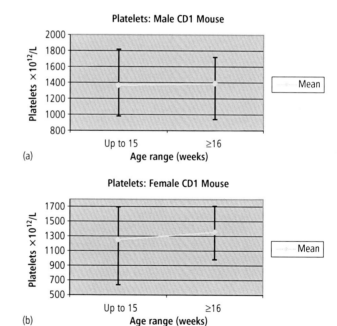

Figure 1.8 Mouse: platelet count (PLT). Male (a) and female (b) animals

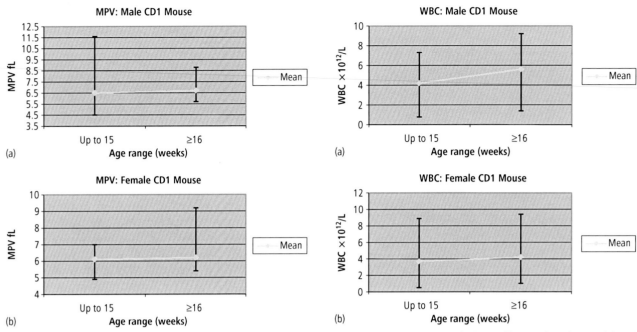

Figure 1.9 Mouse: mean platelet volume (MPV). Male (a) and female (b) animals.

Figure 1.11 Mouse: total white cell count (WBC). Male (a) and female (b) animals.

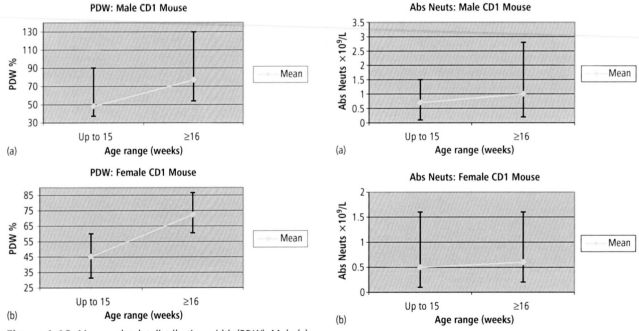

Figure 1.10 Mouse: platelet distribution width (PDW). Male (a) and female (b) animals.

Figure 1.12 Mouse: neutrophil count (Neut). Male (a) and female (b) animals.

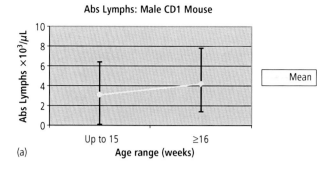

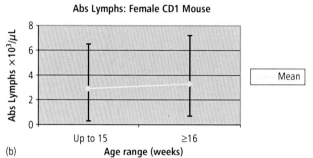

(a)

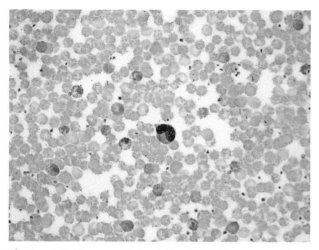

Photo 1.2 Mouse: peripheral blood. Healthy young animal; normal eosinophil and intensely polychromatic cells (×500).

(b)

Figure 1.13 Mouse: lymphocyte count (Lymph). Male (a) and female (b) animals.

The following pictures are stained with modified Wright's stain unless otherwise stated.

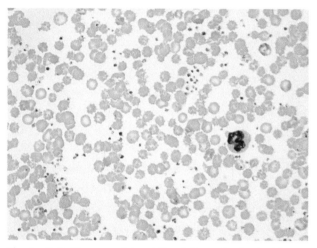

Photo 1.3 Mouse: peripheral blood. Normal animal with age-related crenation and platelet clumps (×500).

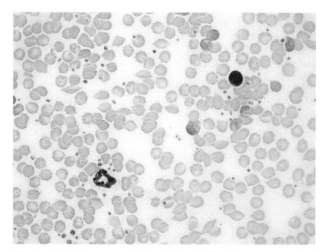

Photo 1.1 Mouse: peripheral blood. Healthy young animal demonstrating a neutrophil, lymphocyte and polychromatic cells (×1000).

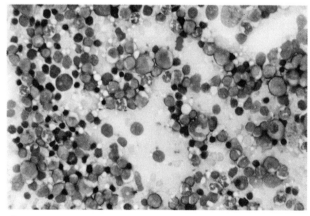

Photo 1.4 Mouse: bone marrow. Normal with good cellularity (×500).

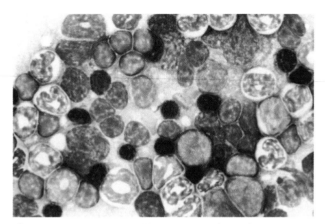

Photo 1.5 Mouse: normal bone marrow (×1000).

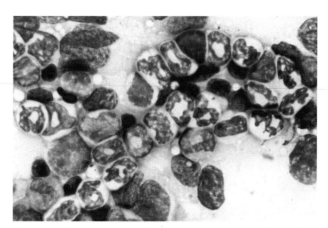

Photo 1.6 Mouse: normal bone marrow. Note annular nucleus in non-segmented neutrophils (×1000).

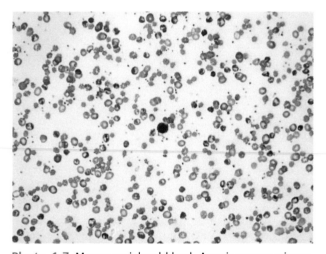

Photo 1.7 Mouse: peripheral blood. Anemic mouse; microcytosis and marked polychromasia (×500).

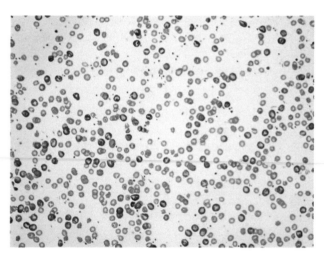

Photo 1.8 Mouse: peripheral blood. Polychromasia with anisocytosis (×500).

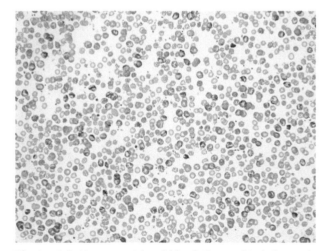

Photo 1.9 Mouse: peripheral blood. Expected polychromasia in a young anemic animal with a typically low white cell count (×500).

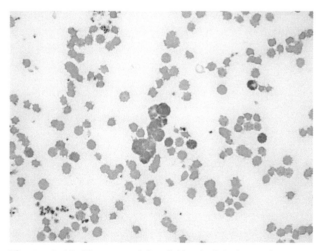

Photo 1.10 Mouse: peripheral blood. Polychromatic aggregates. Care is required as these are sometimes counted as white cells by automated analysers (×1000).

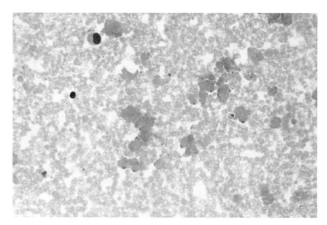

Photo 1.11 Mouse: peripheral blood. Polychromatic aggregates, a common age-related phenomenon in mice (×500).

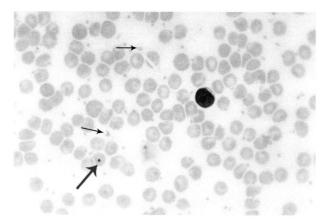

Photo 1.14 Mouse: peripheral blood. Free Heinz bodies (yellow arrow) seen after 24 hours following treatment with azobenzene. These can be confused with platelets (black arrow) by automated analysers. A Howell–Jolly body is indicated by the blue arrow (×1000).

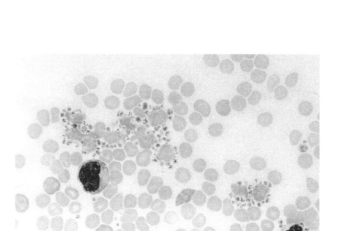

Photo 1.12 Mouse: peripheral blood. Platelet satellitism associated with polychromatic erythrocytes in lymphosarcoma. This unusual phenomenon reflects an affinity between platelets and unspecified determinants on the reticulocyte (×1000).

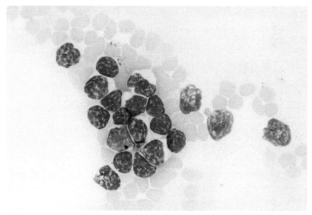

Photo 1.15 Mouse: peripheral blood. Lymphoma: lymphocyte aggregates (×1000).

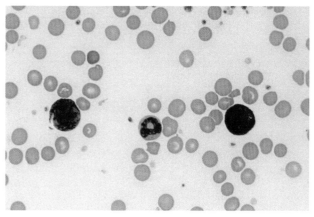

Photo 1.13 Mouse: peripheral blood. Mouse peripheral blood, Basophils with a neutrophil (×1000).

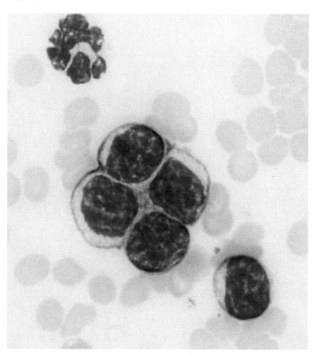

Photo 1.16 Mouse: peripheral blood. Lymphoma: lymphocyte aggregates (×1000).

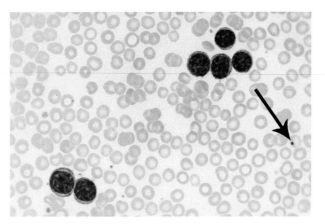

Photo 1.17 Mouse: peripheral blood. Lymphoma: lymphoma aggregates of two to four cells, which affected the automated analysis of this sample. Howell-Jolly body (arrowed). (×1000).

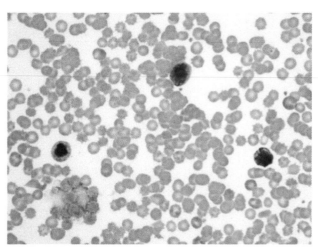

Photo 1.18 Mouse: peripheral blood. Age-degenerated lymphocytes (×1000).

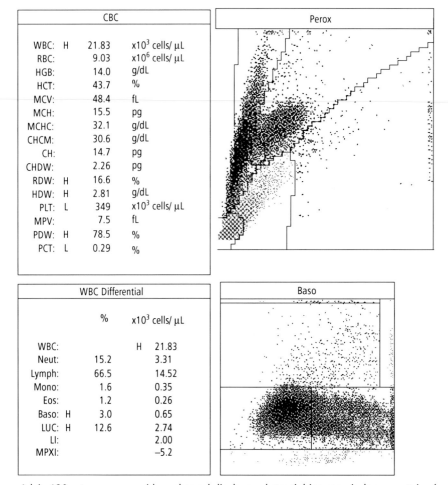

CBC			
WBC:	H	21.83	x10³ cells/ μL
RBC:		9.03	x10⁶ cells/ μL
HGB:		14.0	g/dL
HCT:		43.7	%
MCV:		48.4	fL
MCH:		15.5	pg
MCHC:		32.1	g/dL
CHCM:		30.6	g/dL
CH:		14.7	pg
CHDW:		2.26	pg
RDW:	H	16.6	%
HDW:	H	2.81	g/dL
PLT:	L	349	x10³ cells/ μL
MPV:		7.5	fL
PDW:	H	78.5	%
PCT:	L	0.29	%

WBC Differential		%	x10³ cells/ μL
WBC:			H 21.83
Neut:		15.2	3.31
Lymph:		66.5	14.52
Mono:		1.6	0.35
Eos:		1.2	0.26
Baso:	H	3.0	0.65
LUC:	H	12.6	2.74
LI:			2.00
MPXI:			−5.2

Photo 1.19 Mouse: Advia 120 cytogram, peroxidase channel displays substantial increase in large unstained cells (LUCs).

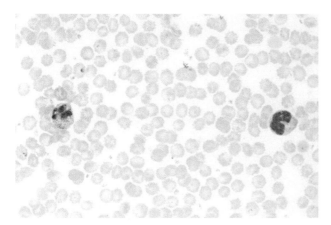

Photo 1.20 Mouse: peripheral blood. Eosinophil metamyelocyte and degenerating basophil (×1000).

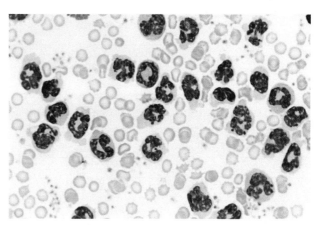

Photo 1.23 Mouse: peripheral blood. Myeloid hyperplasia. This condition is distinct from that of myeloid leukemia in that all the cells present are mature neutrophils; platelet numbers are normal with no nucleated red cells present (×1000).

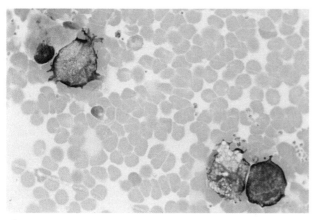

Photo 1.21 Mouse: peripheral blood. Lung dosed. Reactive lymphocyte, metamyelocyte and vacuolated metamyelocyte (×1000).

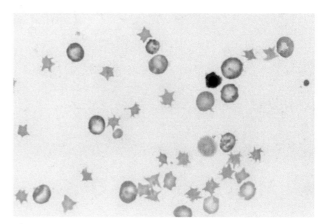

Photo 1.24 Mouse: peripheral blood. Renal failure; marked polychromasia, acanthocytosis with occasional spherocytes, and nucleated red cells (×1000).

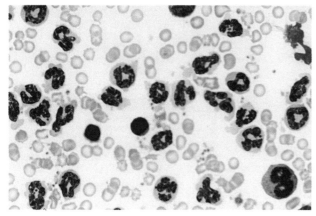

Photo 1.22 Mouse: peripheral blood. Neutrophilia; mouse neutrophils appear to lack stainable granules (×1000).

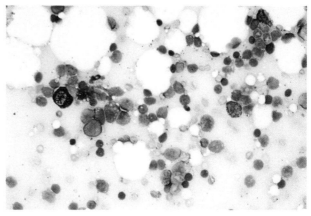

Photo 1.25 Mouse: bone marrow. Aplasia following treatment with busulphan (×1000).

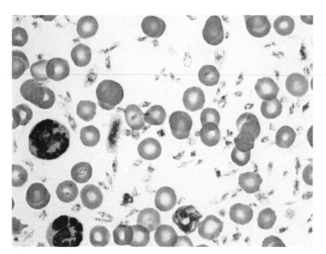

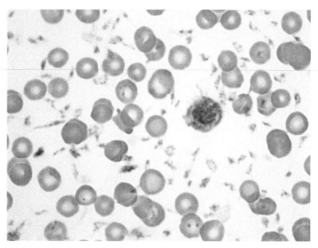

Photo 1.26 Mouse: thrombocythemia (×1000).

Photo 1.27 Mouse: thrombocythemia with giant platelet (×1000).

CBC			
WBC:	H	49.14	x10³ cells/ μL
RBC:		4.43	x10⁶ cells/ μL
HGB:		5.8	g/dL
HCT:		20.9	%
MCV:		47.1	fL
MCH:		13.0	pg
MCHC:		27.7	g/dL
CHCM:		30.0	g/dL
CH:		14.1	pg
CHDW:		2.87	pg
RDW:	H	19.7	%
HDW:	H	3.09	g/dL
PLT:	L	7444	x10³ cells/ μL
MPV:		7.6	fL
PDW:	H	55.2	%
PCT:	L	5.68	%

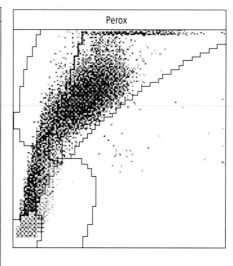

Perox

WBC Differential			
		%	x10³ cells/ μL
WBC:		H	49.18
Neut:	H	78.3	38.51
Lymph:	L	16.8	8.28
Mono:		0.8	0.40
Eos:	L	0.1	0.06
Baso:	H	1.1	0.56
LUC:	H	2.8	1.30
LI:			2.00
MPXI:			8.4

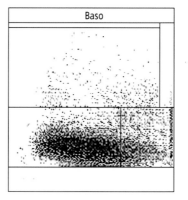

Baso

Photo 1.28 Mouse: thrombocythemia, Advia 120 printout.

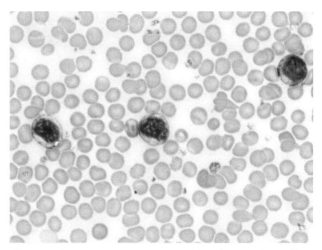

Photo 1.29 Mouse: reactive/atypical lymphocytes (×1000).

CBC			
WBC:	H	370.29	x10³ cells/ µL
RBC:		1.76	x10⁶ cells/ µL
HGB:		3.9	g/dL
HCT:		12.3	%
MCV:		69.5	fL
MCH:		22.2	pg
MCHC:		31.9	g/dL
CHCM:		29.8	g/dL
CH:		20.5	pg
CHDW:		4.45	pg
RDW:	H	23.5	%
HDW:	H	3.95	g/dL
PLT:	L	601	x10³ cells/ µL
MPV:		8.5	fL
PDW:	H	41.7	%
PCT:	L	0.51	%

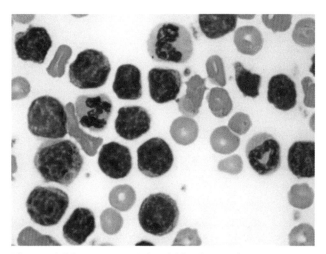

Photo 1.30 Mouse: peripheral blood. Lymphocytic reaction; note the low platelet count (×500).

WBC Differential				
		%	x10³ cells/ µL	
WBC:			H	370.29
Neut:		24.3		90.14
Lymph:	L	54.9		203.31
Mono:		0.6		2.18
Eos:	L	0.1		0.42
Baso:	H	5.7		20.96
LUC:	H	20.0		74.24
LI:				2.65
MPXI:				11.3

Photo 1.32 Same mouse as Photo 1.31. Advia printout.

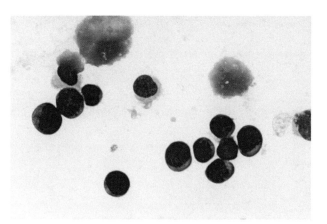

Photo 1.33 Mouse: peripheral blood. Lymphoid reaction with smear cells (×1000).

Photo 1.31 Mouse: peripheral blood. Lymphoma; note the low platelet count (×1000).

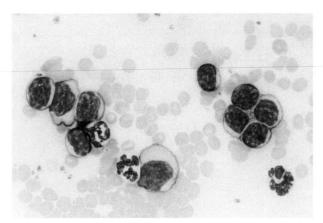

Photo 1.34 Mouse: bone marrow. Lymphoma (×1000).

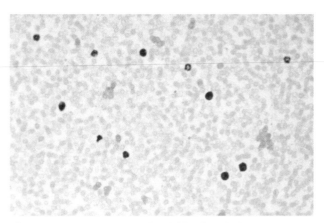

Photo 1.37 Mouse: peripheral blood. Polychromatic aggregates (×500).

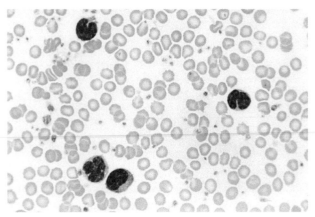

Photo 1.35 Mouse: bone marrow. Lymphoma with cleaved cells (×1000).

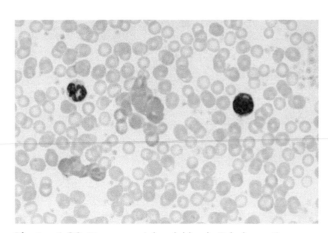

Photo 1.38 Mouse: peripheral blood. Polychromatic aggregates (×500).

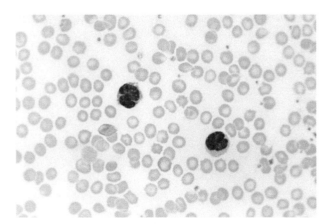

Photo 1.36 Mouse: bone marrow. Lymphoma with cleaved cells. Same animal as Photo 1.35 (×500).

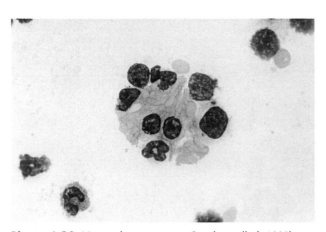

Photo 1.39 Mouse: bone marrow. Gaucher cells (×1000).

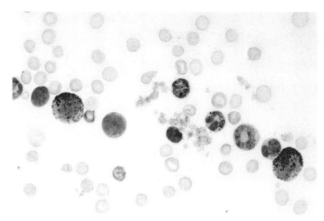

Photo 1.40 Mouse: peripheral blood. Mast cell leukemia; 25% basophils (×1000).

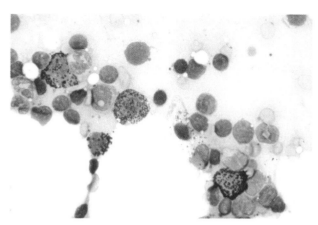

Photo 1.43 Mouse: bone marrow. Mast cell leukaemia; same mouse as Photo 1.40. In spite of bone marrow involvement, only mature forms are present indicating that this is not the primary site of proliferation (×1000).

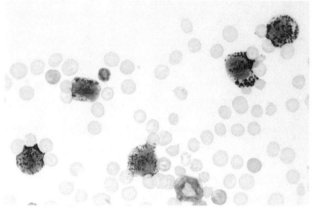

Photo 1.41 Mouse: peripheral blood. Mast cell leukemia; same mouse as Photo 1.40 (×1000).

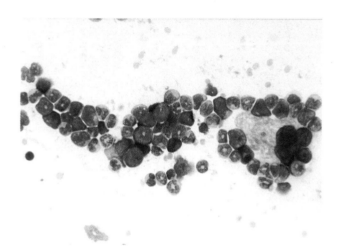

Photo 1.44 Mouse: bone marrow. High M : E ratio (×500).

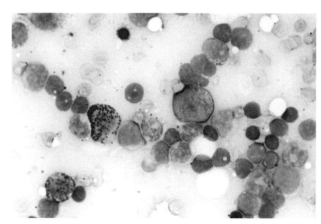

Photo 1.42 Mouse: bone marrow. Mast cell leukemia; same mouse as Photo 1.40 (×1000).

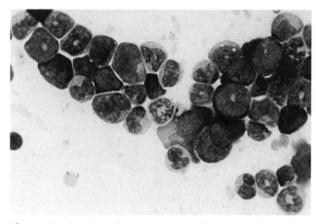

Photo 1.45 Mouse: bone marrow. High M : E ratio (×1000).

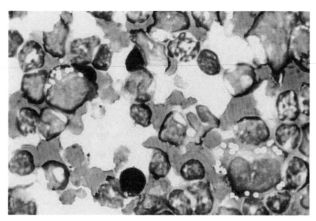

Photo 1.46 Mouse: bone marrow. Vacuolated myeloblasts (×1000).

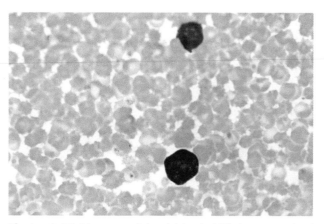

Photo 1.49 Mouse: peripheral blood. 10% large unstained cells shown to be lymphoblasts on the smear (×500).

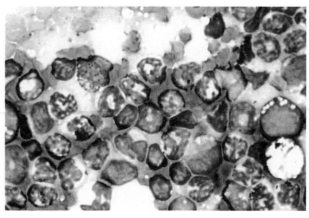

Photo 1.47 Mouse: bone marrow. Vacuolated myeloblasts (×1000).

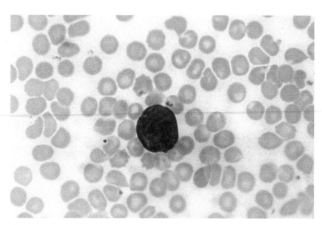

Photo 1.50 Mouse: peripheral blood. 10% large unstained cells shown to be lymphoblasts on the smear (×1000).

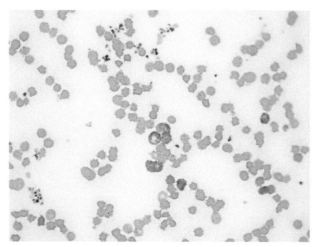

Photo 1.48 Mouse: peripheral blood. Hyperchromic acanthocytes (×500).

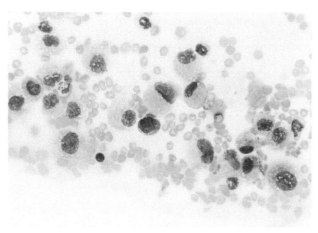

Photo 1.51 Mouse: peripheral blood. Histiocytes following accidental lung dosing (×1000).

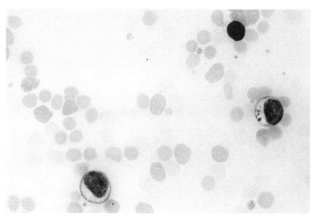

Photo 1.52 Mouse: peripheral blood. Abnormally large granules in lymphocytes (×1000).

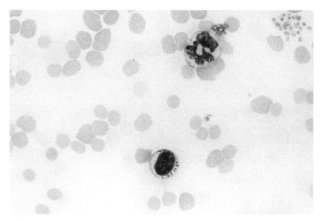

Photo 1.53 Mouse: peripheral blood. Abnormally large granules in lymphocytes (×1000).

HAMSTER

Introduction

Syrian or golden hamsters (*Mesocricetus auratus*) are kept as pets and occasionally employed in toxicological and carcinogenesis research. Blood samples are typically only collected at post mortem due to the difficulty of obtaining a suitable sample. A diurnal variation in number and distribution of leukocytes (principally neutrophils) exists, meaning that cautious data interpretation is necessary.

Blood picture

Red cell counts in this species are generally slightly lower in females than males: MCV values are typically around 70 fL. Reticulocyte counts may be variable in normal animals, and polychromasia is evident on a blood smear.

Neutrophil nuclei may be segmented or unsegmented, and the cytoplasm may contain acidophilic granules leading to the alternative name, heterophils. Eosinophils are unusual, often mono-lobed, and covered by large acidophilic granules which pack the cytoplasm, making the cell relatively easy to distinguish from neutrophils/heterophils.

Platelet numbers in hamsters are high compared to those of humans, low compared to those of other rodents, averaging around 350–400 × 10^3/μL, and are lower during hibernation.

Reference range data are not available from our laboratories due to the low numbers of this species used.

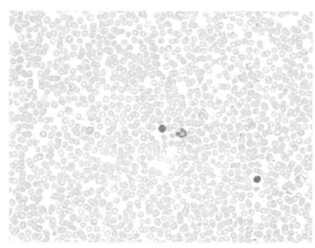

Photo 1.54 Hamster: peripheral blood. A neutrophil, two lymphocytes and polychromasia (×500).

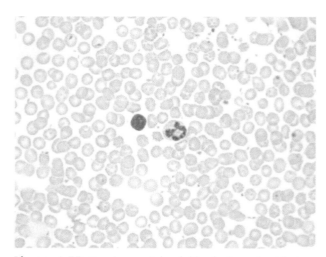

Photo 1.55 Hamster: peripheral blood. A neutrophil, lymphocyte and polychromasia (×500).

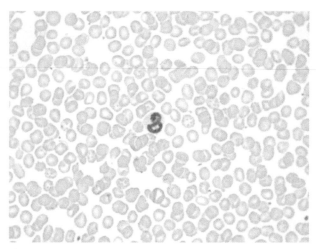

Photo 1.56 Hamster: peripheral blood. A neutrophil, and poly-chromasia (×500).

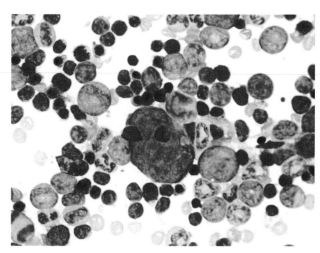

Photo 1.59 Hamster: normal bone marrow (×500).

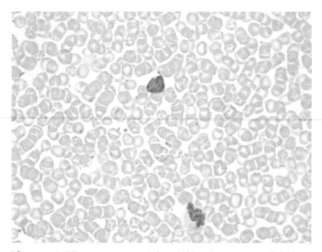

Photo 1.57 Hamster: peripheral blood. A neutrophil, lymphocyte and polychromasia (×500).

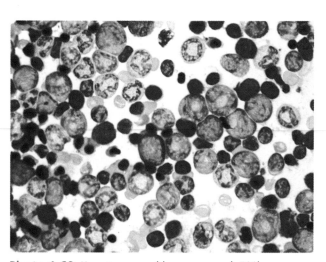

Photo 1.60 Hamster: normal bone marrow (×500).

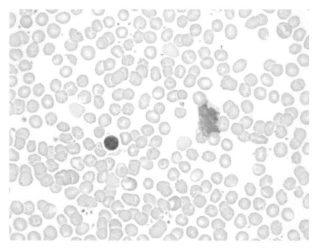

Photo 1.58 Hamster: peripheral blood. Small and large lymphocytes, polychromasia and target cells (×1000).

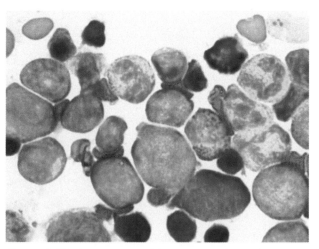

Photo 1.61 Hamster: normal bone marrow (×1000).

GUINEA PIG

Introduction

The guinea pig (*Cavia porcellus*) is kept as a pet and widely employed in immunotoxicological investigations.

Blood picture

There are significant sex differences in most red cell parameters in the adult animal with female RBC values up to 20% lower than age-matched males. The red cell of the female is larger than that of the male, typically around 82 fL[6].

The leukocyte population shows great variability between individuals with a number of distinctive features. The neutrophil nucleus tends to be highly lobulated and polymorphous and the acidophilic granules of the cytoplasm, smaller than those of eosinophils, promote the term "pseudo-eosinophil". The eosinophil, which is customarily mono-lobed, is covered by large acidophilic granules which pack the cytoplasm making the cell relatively easy to distinguish from the pseudo-eosinophil. Basophils are rare. Monocytes are the largest leukocyte in the circulation; compared to lymphocytes they are larger and have a darker, more abundant cytoplasm, often with an oval nucleus.

Large lymphocytes often containing variably sized azurophilic granules. A unique feature of guinea pig lymphocytes is the occurrence of a number of "T" lymphocytes which have single, or rarely multiple, inclusion bodies consisting of mucopolysaccharide, staining diffusely red with reddish granulation. Known as Foa–Kurloff cells, they possibly function as natural killer cells[7].

Platelet counts in guinea pigs are higher than in humans but low compared to other rodents, with values around $500 \times 10^3/\mu L$; they are quite small and spindle shaped.

Reference range data are not available from our laboratories due to the low numbers of this species used.

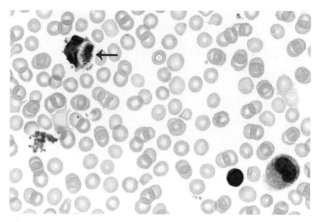

Photo 1.63 Guinea pig: peripheral blood. Histiocyte or monocyte, lymphocyte and a lymphocyte with a large mucopolysaccharide inclusion (Foa–Kurloff body, arrow) (×1000).

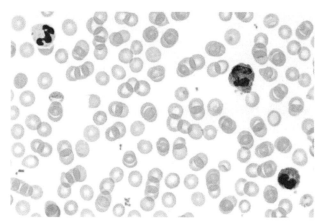

Photo 1.62 Guinea pig: peripheral blood. Neutrophil, two basophils and basophilic stippling in a red cell (×1000).

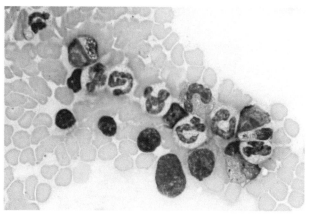

Photo 1.64 Guinea pig: peripheral blood. Foa–Kurloff body in two lymphocytes in the tail end of the smear (×1000).

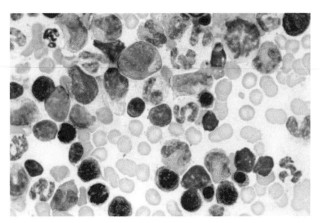

Photo 1.65 Guinea pig: bone marrow. Normal (×1000).

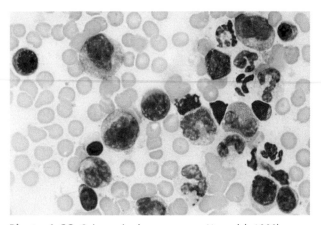

Photo 1.66 Guinea pig: bone marrow. Normal (×1000).

RAT – SPRAGUE DAWLEY (SD)/HAN WISTAR (HW)

Introduction

Many strains of rat (*Rattus norvegicus*) are kept as pets, used in research and employed in preclinical studies. The descriptions detailed here are based on our experiences with Sprague Dawley and Han Wistar rats, but most comments are equally applicable to most other strains.

Blood picture

Erythrocyte counts tend to be high in comparison to those of larger mammals due to rats' high metabolic rate, typically in the range $6.8–10.05 \times 10^6$ cells/µL. Hemoglobin values vary with strain and are determined by sex, age and health. The diameter of the erythrocyte in the rat varies between 5.7 and 7 µm, depending on its maturity[8]. MCH values (typically of 16–21 pg) reflect the small size of red cells in this species, whilst the MCHC tends to be close to 33.5 g/dL in fresh samples from mature animals.

RDW and HDW reflect the variability of the distribution of the population of red cells, normal values in rats tending to be similar to those in humans and within the ranges RDW = 9.3–27.6% and HDW = 1.64–3.33 g/dL. Erythrocytes from normal healthy animals therefore show marked anisocytosis and poikilocytosis, becoming noticeably more marked with time after sample collection. Typically, crenation becomes evident 20–30 minutes after sampling, the severity increasing with time until spherocytes, echinocytes and/or sphero-echinocytes predominate. Automated cell counters that measure intra-erythrocyte hemoglobin concentration and distribution (CHCM and RDW) may detect polychromatic erythrocytes that are resistant to these changes.

At birth, almost all erythrocytes are reticulocytes, falling near to adult levels (0.2–4.0%) by ~40 days, appropriately reflected in the degree of polychromasia. Occasional normoblasts are often seen in normal healthy animals.

There is a great variation in total leukocyte count and differential distribution due to the excitable nature of the animals, the site of sampling and normal diurnal variations.

Lymphocytes constitute the majority white cell population in peripheral blood and are seen as a relatively homogeneous population in a healthy subject. Both large and small lymphocytes are present, the former approximating to the size of normal neutrophils and sometimes containing large, dark-staining azurophilic granules. The nuclei of the latter are slightly larger than erythrocytes.

Neutrophils are the next most numerous leukocyte. Nuclear lobulation distribution shows a slight right shift in comparison with human neutrophils. The formation of lobes in the granulocytes of rats (and other rodents) is preceded by the development of an annular nucleus. This phenomenon first becomes apparent in the promyelocyte stage in bone marrow, metamyelocytes appearing uniformly "doughnut shaped". This ring structure may not be entirely lost even in the most mature neutrophils, so some cells possess nuclei in figure-of-eight conformation. It is interesting to note, however, that this annular structure tends to be lost in chronic myeloid leukemia (CML).

Monocytes are normally present only in low numbers in peripheral blood in healthy animals, but can constitute up to 6% of the differential. Nuclei tend to be variable in shape; the cytoplasm is basophilic, often vacuolated and may contain azurophilic granules.

Eosinophils are also normally present only in low numbers in peripheral blood in healthy animals. They are generally larger than neutrophils with small, round, strongly acidophilic granules which fill the cytoplasm. Immature nuclei often appear "doughnut shaped".

Care must be taken when assessing data from stored samples analysed on automated analysers as degraded neutrophils may be mistaken for monocytes and eosinophils and the differential may be inaccurate. Microscopic evaluation is therefore critical to ensuring the integrity of these counts.

Basophils are uncommon, or absent, in rat blood preparations in some strains. Bone marrow mast cells similarly vary in their incidence, pigmented strains having a higher incidence than albino animals.

Large unstained cells (LUCs) constitute around 5% of a normal population of circulating white blood cells, and reflect the same situation as in other species, i.e. increases are due to reactive, activated or atypical lymphocytes, or mononuclear cells.

Platelet numbers vary greatly in the literature[6,9,10,11], but are greater in number with smaller individual volume than human platelets, with values in our laboratories for MPV of 5.7–10.1 fL. Platelet counts, volume estimations and population statistics may be compromised by degranulation, clumping of platelets and/or partial clotting of the sample. Platelet count validity must be considered very carefully in the light of microscopic examination of the blood smear.

Typical ranges (Siemens Advia 120)

The following reference range data are taken from our own laboratories. These data are specifically obtained

from the HW strain, but SD data are available and very similar. Due to the low numbers of monocytes, eosinophils, basophils and large unstained cells present in peripheral blood, these data are not expressed here.

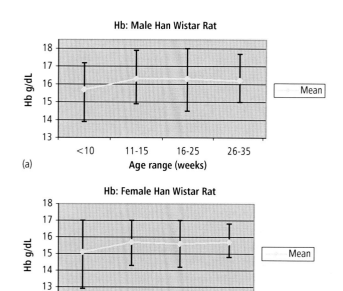

Figure 1.14 Rat: hemoglobin (Hb). Male (a) and female (b) animals.

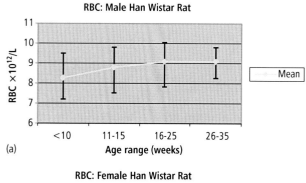

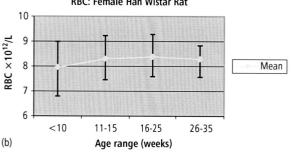

Figure 1.15 Rat: red cell count (RBC). Male (a) and female (b) animals.

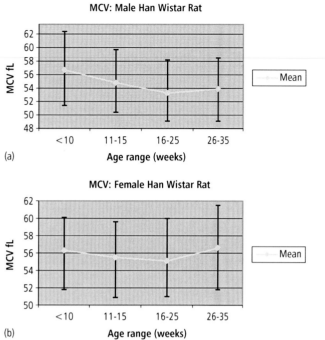

(a)

(b)

Figure 1.16 Rat: mean cell volume (MCV). Male (a) and female (b) animals.

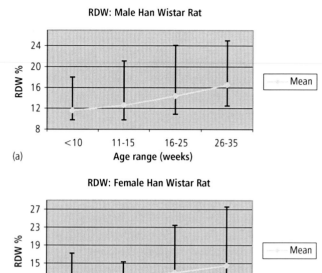

(a)

(b)

Figure 1.18 Rat: red cell distribution width (RDW). Male (a) and female (b) animals.

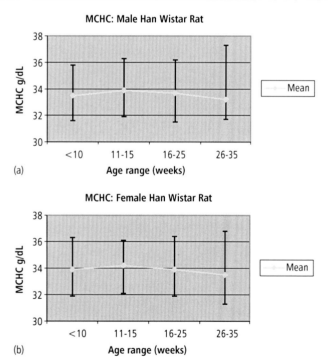

(a)

(b)

Figure 1.17 Rat: mean cell hemoglobin concentration (MCHC). Male (a) and female (b) animals.

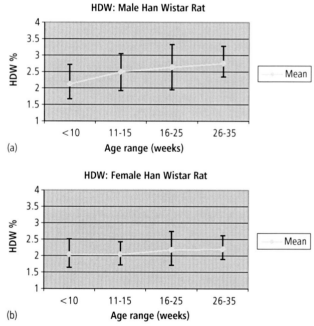

(a)

(b)

Figure 1.19 Rat: hemoglobin distribution width (HDW). Male (a) and female (b) animals.

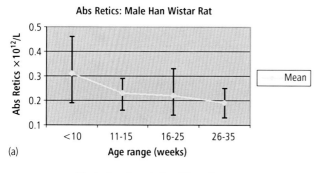

(a)

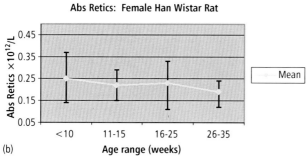

(b)

Figure 1.20 Rat: absolute reticulocyte count (Retic Abs). Male (a) and female (b) animals.

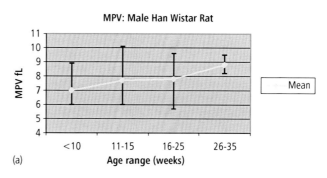

(a)

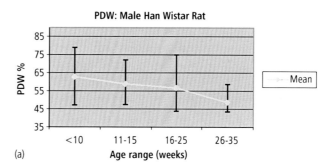

(b)

Figure 1.22 Rat: mean platelet volume (MPV). Male (a) and female (b) animals.

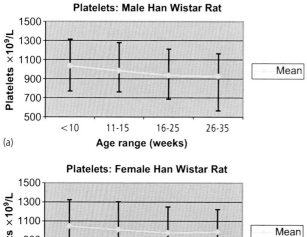

(a)

(b)

Figure 1.21 Rat: platelet count (PLT). Male (a) and female (b) animals.

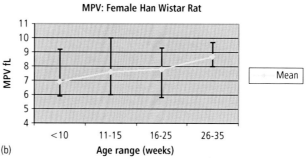

(a)

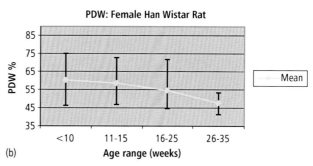

(b)

Figure 1.23 Rat: platelet distribution width (PDW). Male (a) and female (b) animals.

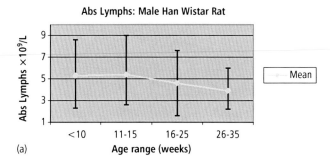

(a)

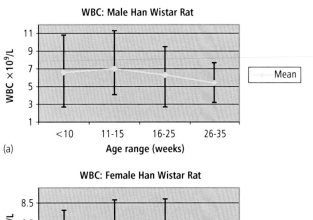

(b)

Figure 1.24 Rat: total white cell count (WBC). Male (a) and female (b) animals.

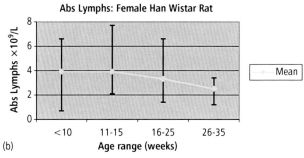

(a)

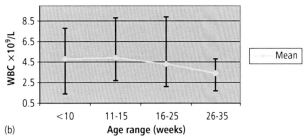

(b)

Figure 1.26 Rat: lymphocyte count (Lymph). Male (a) and female (b) animals.

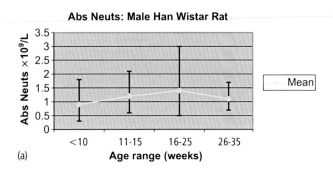

(a)

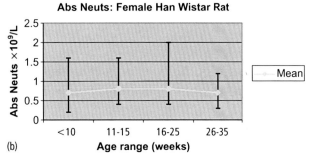

(b)

Figure 1.25 Rat: neutrophil count (Neut). Male (a) and female (b) animals.

The following pictures are stained with modified Wright's stain unless otherwise stated.

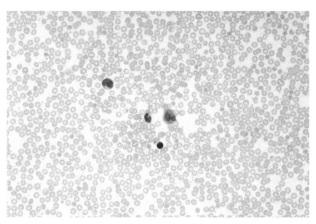

Photo 1.67 Rat: peripheral blood. Neutrophil, lymphocyte, monocyte and eosinophil (×500).

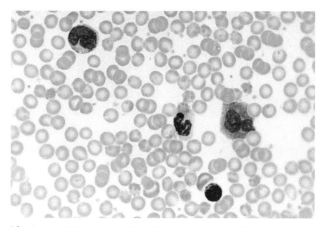

Photo 1.68 Rat: peripheral blood. Neutrophil, lymphocyte, monocyte and eosinophil (×1000).

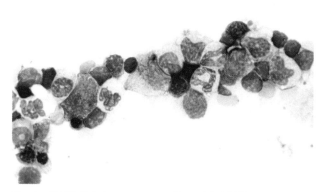

Photo 1.71 Rat: bone marrow. Normal (×1000).

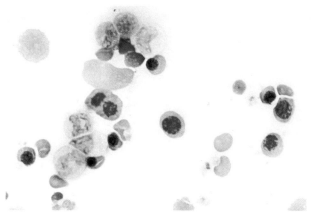

Photo 1.69 Rat: bone marrow. Metamyelocytes, intermediate and late erythroblasts and a dividing erythroblast (×1000).

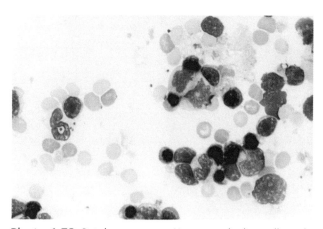

Photo 1.72 Rat: bone marrow. Note some broken cells probably from the preparation process (×1000).

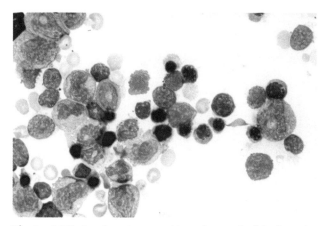

Photo 1.70 Rat: bone marrow. Normal; note the "ring" myelocytes (×1000).

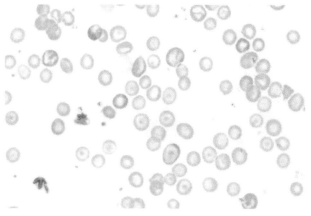

Photo 1.73 Rat: peripheral blood. Target cells (×1000).

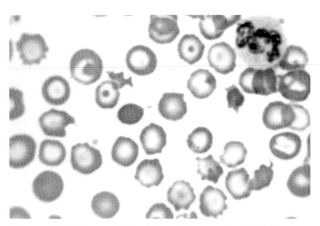

Photo 1.74 Rat: peripheral blood. Target cells (×1200).

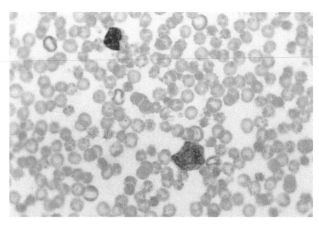

Photo 1.77 Rat: peripheral blood. Eosinophil and lymphocyte (×1000).

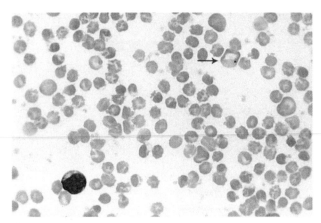

Photo 1.75 Rat: peripheral blood. Early lymphocyte with hyperchromia, polychromasia, crenation and a Howell–Jolly body (arrow) (×1000).

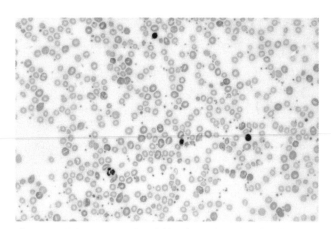

Photo 1.78 Rat: peripheral blood. Nucleated red cells, polychromasia and anisocytosis (×500).

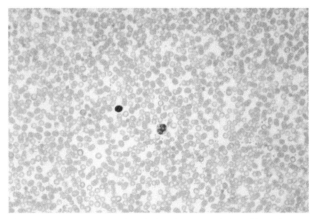

Photo 1.76 Rat: peripheral blood. Neutrophil and lymphocyte (×500).

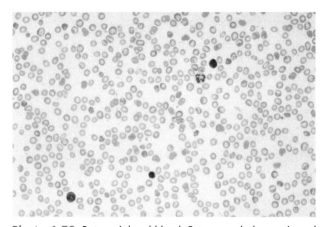

Photo 1.79 Rat: peripheral blood. Extreme polychromasia and low platelet count (×500).

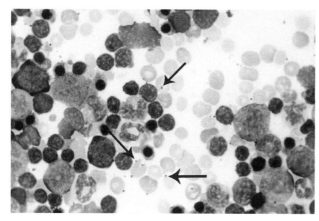

Photo 1.80 Rat: bone marrow. Howell–Jolly bodies (arrowed) (×1000).

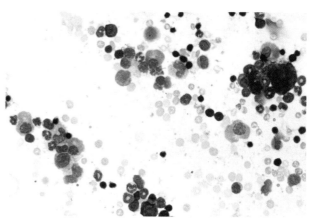

Photo 1.83 Rat: bone marrow. Plasma cell excess (×500).

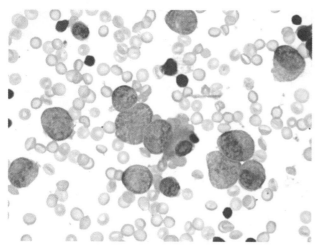

Photo 1.81 Rat: bone marrow. Leukemoid reaction; myeloblast hyperplasia (×1000).

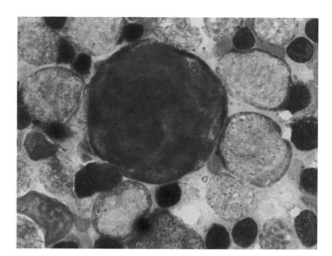

Photo 1.84 Rat: bone marrow. Reticulum cell (×1000).

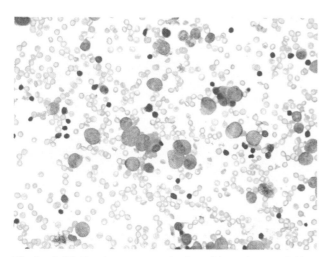

Photo 1.82 Rat: bone marrow. Leukemoid reaction; myeloblast hyperplasia (MGG stain) (×500).

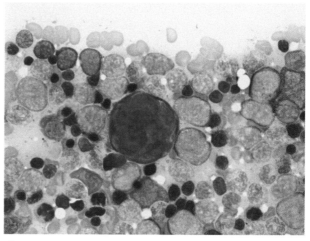

Photo 1.85 Rat: bone marrow. Reticulum cell (×1000).

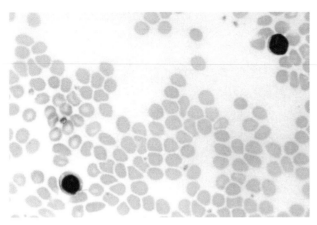

Photo 1.86 Rat: peripheral blood. Vacuolated lymphocyte (×500).

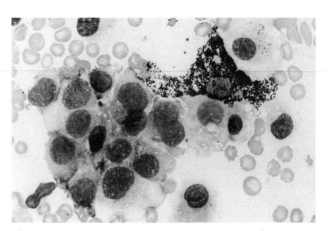

Photo 1.89 Rat: peripheral blood. HLS. Clump of histiocytes with a mast cell in association with neoplastic cells (×1000).

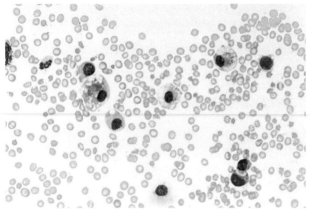

Photo 1.87 Rat: peripheral blood. Histiocytic lymphosarcoma (HLS); histiocytes (large monocytoid cells with foamy cytoplasm) (×500)

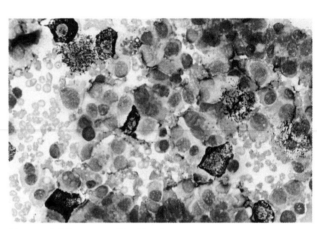

Photo 1.90 Rat: cardiac blood. HLS same case as Photo 1.87. A large clump of histiocytes from the tail of the smear. Many mast cells were present indicating a co-existing proliferation although it should be noted that samples obtained from the peritoneal cavity are often contaminated with mast cells which are not present in the peripheral circulation (×500).

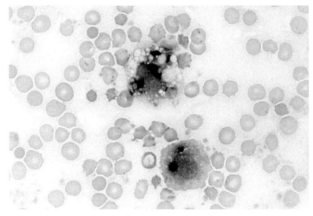

Photo 1.88 Rat: peripheral blood. HLS; dual esterase staining (×1000).

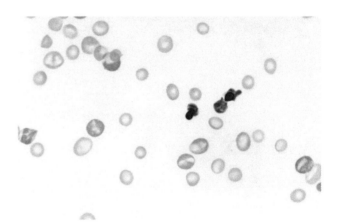

Photo 1.91 Rat: peripheral blood. Polychromasia with pyknotic nucleated red cells (×500).

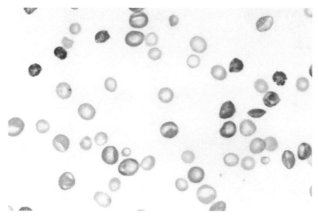

Photo 1.92 Rat: peripheral blood. Polychromasia, anisocytosis, with a Howell–Jolly body (×1000).

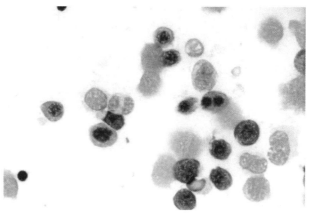

Photo 1.95 Rat: bone marrow. Normoblasts and mitotic cell. Note the excessive cell debris believed to be of myeloid origin (×1000).

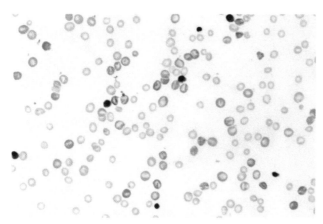

Photo 1.93 Rat: peripheral blood. Extreme polychromasia and anisocytosis with many pyknotic nucleated red cells (×500).

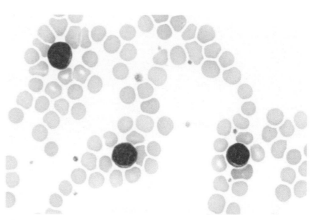

Photo 1.96 Rat: peripheral blood. Lymphoblasts (×1000).

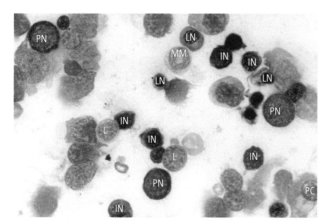

Photo 1.94 Rat: bone marrow. Normoblast proliferation. Key: PN, pronormoblast; IN, intermediate normoblast; LN, late normoblast; MM, myelocyte; L, lymphocyte (×1000).

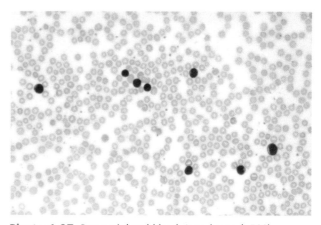

Photo 1.97 Rat: peripheral blood. Lymphoma (×500).

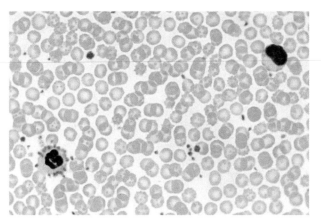

Photo 1.98 Rat: peripheral blood. Lymphoma; neutrophil with platelet satellitism (×1000).

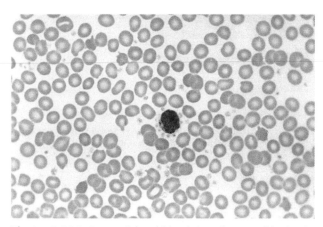

Photo 1.101 Rat: peripheral blood. Lymphocyte with platelet satellitism (×1000).

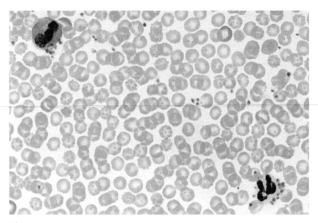

Photo 1.99 Rat: peripheral blood. Neutrophils with platelet satellitism (×1000).

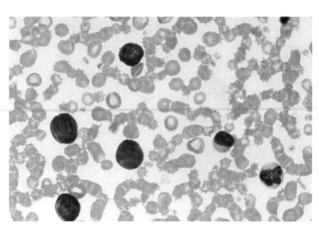

Photo 1.102 Rat: peripheral blood. Lymphoblasts (×1000).

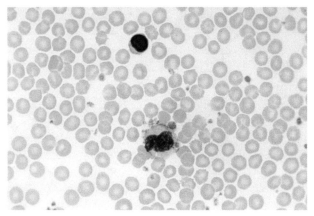

Photo 1.100 Rat: peripheral blood. Lymphocyte and neutrophil with platelet satellitism (×1000).

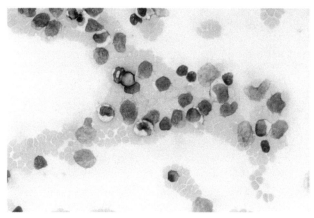

Photo 1.103 Rat: peripheral blood. Lymphoma. Thin end of a smear (×1000).

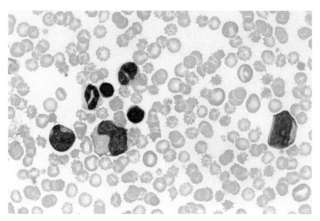

Photo 1.104 Rat: peripheral blood. Lymphoma with marked red cell crenation (×1000)

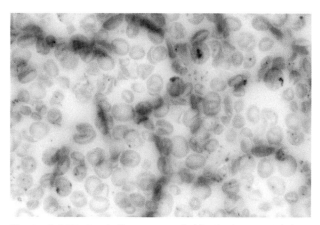

Photo 1.107 Rat: buffy coat. Lymphoblastic picture. Acid phosphatase stain (×500).

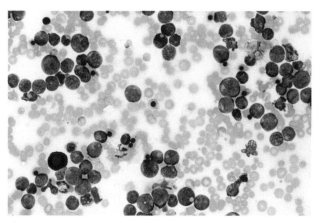

Photo 1.105 Rat: peripheral blood. Lymphoma with large number of lymphoblasts and numerous nucleated red cells (×500).

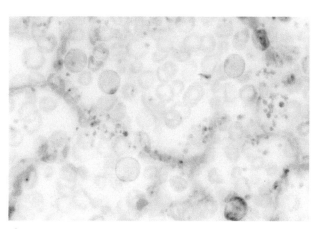

Photo 1.108 Rat: buffy coat. Lymphoblastic picture. Dual esterase stain (×500).

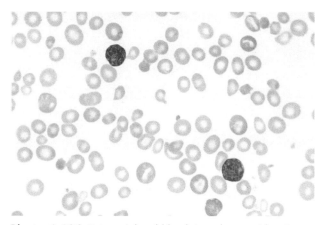

Photo 1.106 Rat: peripheral blood. Lymphoma with anisopoikilocytosis (×1000).

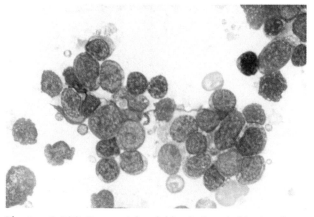

Photo 1.109 Rat: peripheral blood. Lymphoblastic picture (×1000).

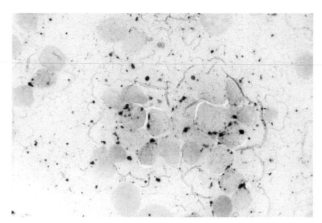

Photo 1.110 Rat: peripheral blood. Lymphoblastic picture. Alkaline phosphatase stain (×1000).

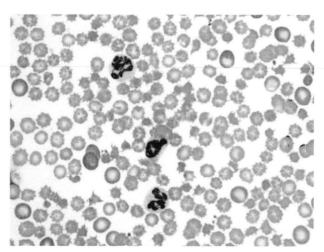

Photo 1.113 Rat: peripheral blood. Neutrophil hypersegmentation (×500).

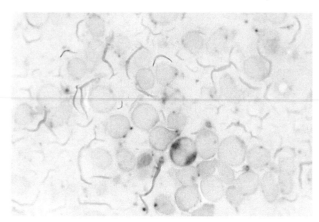

Photo 1.111 Rat: peripheral blood. Lymphoblastic picture. Alpha-naphthyl acetate esterase stain (ANAE, brown) (×1000).

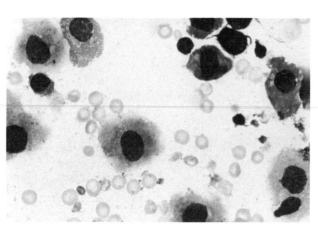

Photo 1.114 Rat: bone marrow. Histiocytic lymphosarcoma with large foamy monocytoid histiocytes (×1000).

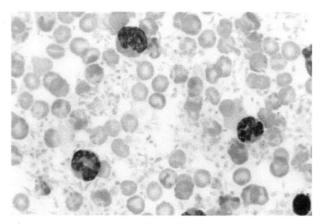

Photo 1.112 Rat: peripheral blood cytospin preparation. 33.6% eosinophils with a high platelet count (×1000).

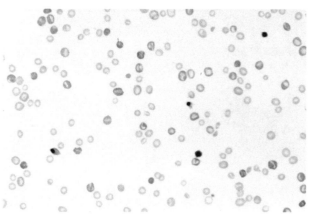

Photo 1.115 Rat: peripheral blood. Hb 2.6 g/dL. Extreme polychromasia and nucleated red cells (×500).

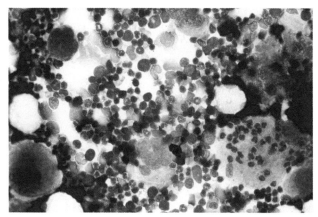

Photo 1.116 Rat: bone marrow. Megakaryocytes showing emperipolesis or phagocytosis in an animal treated with an inhibitor of androgen synthesis. Neutrophils appear not only to be passing through the cytoplasm, but actively congregating inside megakaryocytes (×500).

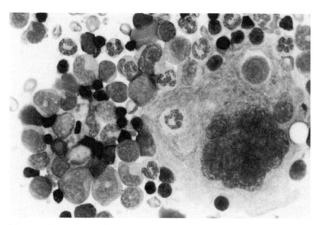

Photo 1.119 Rat: bone marrow. Phagocytosis or emperipolesis in an animal treated with an inhibitor of androgen synthesis. Same animal as Photo 1.116 (×1000).

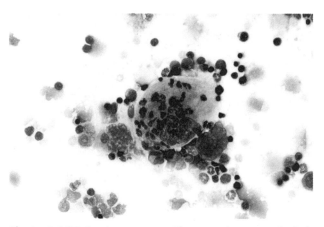

Photo 1.117 Rat: bone marrow. Phagocytosis or emperipolesis in an animal treated with an inhibitor of androgen synthesis. Same animal as Photo 1.116 (×500).

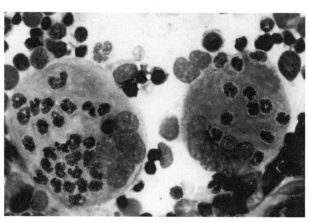

Photo 1.120 Rat: bone marrow. Phagocytosis or emperipolesis in an animal treated with an inhibitor of androgen synthesis. Same animal as Photo 1.116 (×1000).

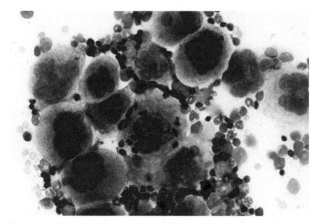

Photo 1.118 Rat: bone marrow. Phagocytosis or emperipolesis in an animal treated with an inhibitor of androgen synthesis. Same animal as Photo 1.116 (×500).

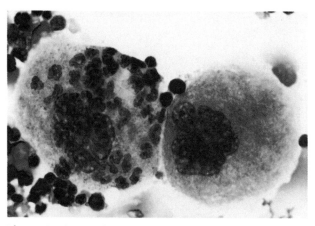

Photo 1.121 Rat: bone marrow. Phagocytosis or emperipolesis in an animal treated with an inhibitor of androgen synthesis. Same animal as Photo 1.116 (×1000).

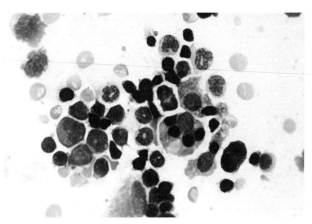

Photo 1.122 Rat: bone marrow. Erythrophagocytosis of normoblasts (×1000).

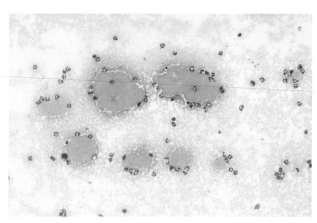

Photo 1.125 Rat: peripheral blood. Neutrophil/globular cluster aggregates. Same animal as Photo 1.124 (×500).

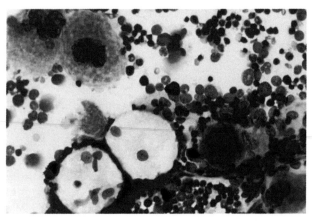

Photo 1.123 Rat: bone marrow. Vacuolated macrophages and mast cells. Same animal as Photo 1.122 (×1000).

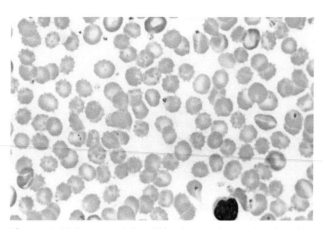

Photo 1.126 Rat: peripheral blood. Acanthocytosis induced by a biological response modifier (BRM) (×1000).

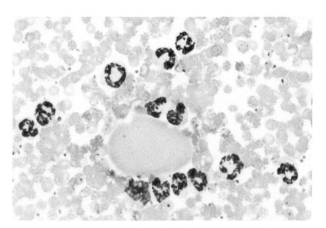

Photo 1.124 Rat: peripheral blood. Precipitation of globular material and associated neutrophilia. This unusual phenomenon appeared at room temperature and may reflect an interaction between the administered compound and plasma proteins (×1000).

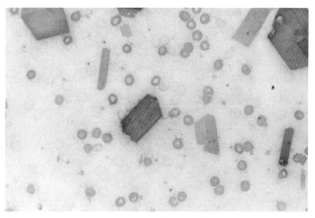

Photo 1.127 Rat: peripheral blood. Artifact Hb crystals caused by partial freezing of the sample (×1000).

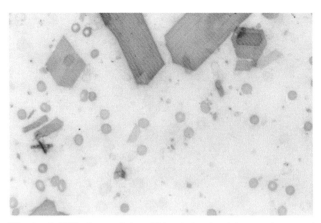

Photo 1.128 Rat: peripheral blood. Artefact Hb crystals caused by partial freezing of the sample (×1000).

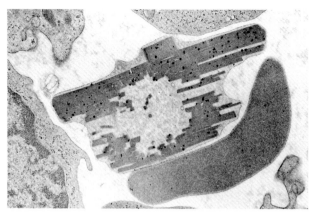

Photo 1.131 Rat: peripheral blood. Intra-erythrocytic Hb crystals (electron microscope (EM)).

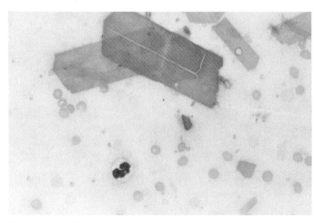

Photo 1.129 Rat: peripheral blood. Artefact Hb crystals caused by partial freezing of the sample (×1000).

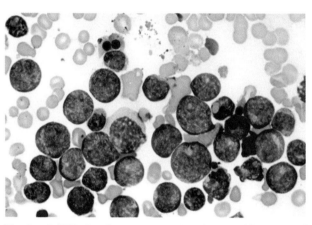

Photo 1.132 Rat: bone marrow. Lymphoma with suspected erythrophagocytosis (×1000).

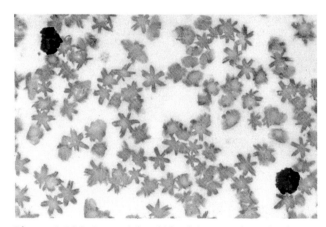

Photo 1.130 Rat: peripheral blood. Intra-erythrocytic Hb crystals (×500).

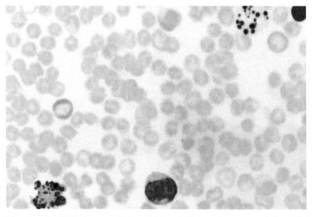

Photo 1.133 Rat: peripheral blood. Pyknotic neutrophil nuclei following treatment with a novel anti-cancer agent (×500).

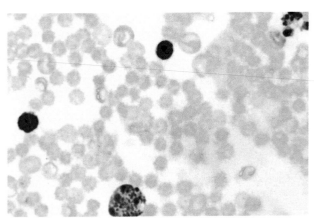

Photo 1.134 Rat: peripheral blood. Pyknotic neutrophil nuclei following treatment with a novel anti-cancer agent: same animal as Photo 1.133 (×500).

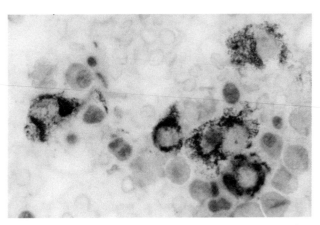

Photo 1.137 Rat: bone marrow. Histiocytes. Same animal as Photo 1.135 stained with esterase (×1000).

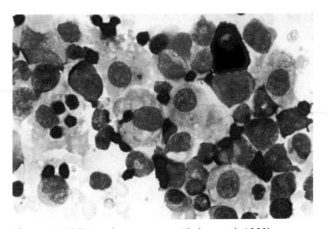

Photo 1.135 Rat: bone marrow. Histiocytes (×1000).

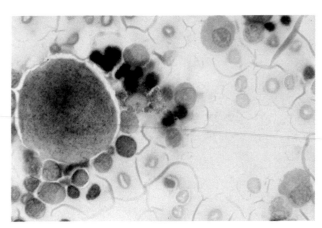

Photo 1.138 Rat: bone marrow. Histiocytes. Same animal as Photo 1.135 stained with esterase (×1000).

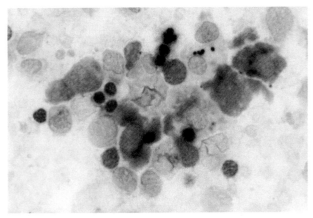

Photo 1.136 Rat: bone marrow. Histiocytes. Same animal as Photo 1.135 stained with esterase (×1000).

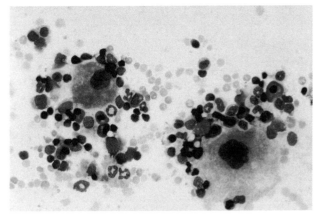

Photo 1.139 Rat: bone marrow. Plasma cells and megakaryocytes (×500).

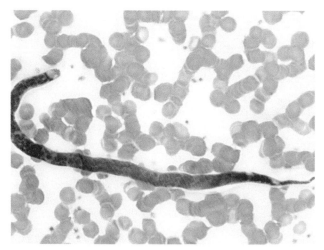

Photo 1.140 Rat: peripheral blood. Microfilaria (×1000).

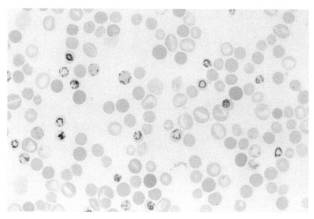

Photo 1.143 Rat: peripheral blood. 20-day-old rat, reticulocytosis. New methylene blue stain (×500).

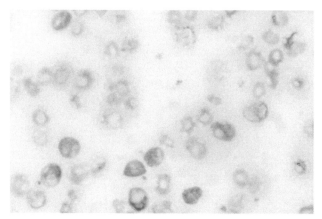

Photo 1.141 Rat: peripheral blood. Dysplastic red cells caused by a novel anti-cancer drug (×1000).

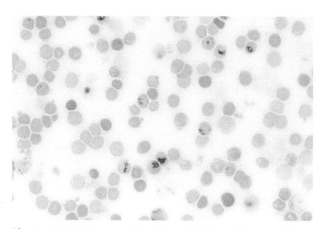

Photo 1.144 Rat: peripheral blood. 30-day-old rat, reticulocytosis. New methylene blue stain (×500).

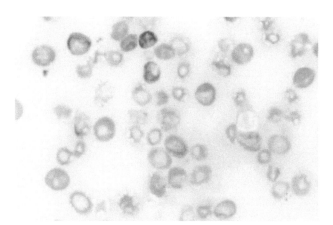

Photo 1.142 Rat: peripheral blood. Dysplastic red cells caused by a novel anti-cancer drug (×1000).

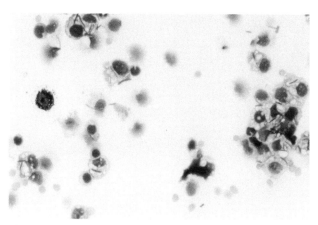

Photo 1.145 Rat: peritoneal wash. Mast cells and bacteria (×500).

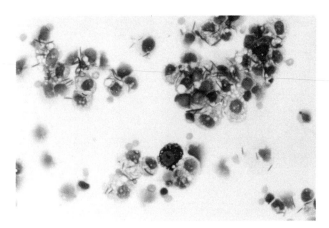

Photo 1.146 Rat: peritoneal wash. Same animal as Photo 1.145 (×500).

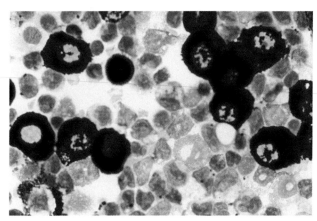

Photo 1.147 Rat: peritoneal cytospin. Displaying numerous mast cells (×1000).

References

1. Mueller P, Diamond J (2001). Metabolic rate and environmental productivity: well-provisioned animals evolved to run and idle fast. *Proc Natl Acad Sci USA* 98(22): 12550–12554.
2. Plata EJ, Murphy WH (1972). Growth and haematologic properties of the BALB/wm strain of inbred mice. *Lab Anim Sci* 22:701–720.
3. Schermer S (1967). *The Blood Morphology of Laboratory Animals*. Philadelphia: FA Davis.
4. Harrison SD, *et al.* (1978). Haematology and clinical chemistry reference values. *Cancer Res* 38: 2636–2639.
5. Harkness JE, Wagner JE (1995). *The Biology and Medicine of Rabbits and Rodents (4th edn)*. Baltimore: Williams and Wilkins.
6. Mitruka BJ, Rawnsley HM (1981). *Clinical Biochemical and Haematological Reference Values in Normal Experimental Animals and Normal Humans (2nd edn)*. New York: Masson.
7. Pouliot N, Maghni K, Blanchette F, *et al.* (1996). Natural killer and lectin-dependent cytotoxic activities of Kurloff cells: target cell selectivity, conjugate formation, and Ca++ dependency. *Inflammation* 20: 647–671.
8. Feldman BF, Zinkl JG, Jain NC (eds) (2010). *Schalm's Veterinary Hematology (6th edn)*. Baltimore: Lippincott Williams & Wilkins.
9. Conybeare G, Leslie GB, *et al.* (1988). An improved simple technique for the collection of blood samples from rats and mice. *Lab Anim* 22: 177–182.
10. Leonard R, Ruben Z (1986). Haematology reference values for peripheral blood of laboratory rats. *Lab Anim Sci* 36: 277–281.
11. Levin J, Ebbe S (1994). Letter; comment – Why are recently published platelet counts in normal mice so low? *Blood* 83(12): 3829–3831.

2

Rabbit

Introduction

Rabbits are popular pets and are the animals of choice in teratological studies, New Zealand white (*Oryctolagus cuniculus*) being most popular. Sex and strain differences are minimal in these animals, and there are only minimal age-related effects. By contrast, wild animals, e.g. European brown hares (*Lepus europaeus*), have red cell counts and hemoglobin values higher in adults than in young animals[1].

Blood picture

Wild rabbits have a smaller mean cell volume than domesticated animals. Reticulocytes are quite common in very young rabbits, and small rouleaux frequently form in the blood film. Marked anisocytosis is a prominent feature of rabbit erythrocytes and they may exhibit a "thorn apple" appearance.

Leukocyte counts exhibit diurnal rhythms, and variations with age, gender, breed and diet make data interpretation problematic. Neutrophil:lymphocyte ratios tend to diminish from 1:2 to 1:1 as rabbits age from 3 months to 1 year, and data interpretation is made more difficult as this ratio can be affected by stress[2].

Neutrophils are distinctive and can be mistaken for eosinophils as the cytoplasm is strongly granulated with two types of red-staining granules: there is a fine hazy dusting of small diffuse granules giving a pink appearance to the cytoplasm overlaid with a scattering of large acidophilic and red granules. The true eosinophil is characterised by many intensely acidophilic large granules packing the cytoplasm of the cell and a horseshoe-shaped or bi-lobed nucleus. The rabbit is unique amongst laboratory animals as the population of peripheral blood basophils is quite substantial, sometimes up to 10%.

Rabbits may display the Pelger–Huët anomaly in which the nucleus of granulocytes, especially that of the neutrophil, does not mature to the segmented form resulting in an apparent left shift in adult neutrophils. This condition may occur in otherwise healthy individuals, although it may also be seen as a lethal homozygote form or a benign heterozygote condition.

Hematological disorders are otherwise uncommon in rabbits.

There is a wide variety of platelet counts reported in the literature[3,4,5,6]. Our own experience shows that platelet activation and consequent clumping is inherent in peripheral blood collection and may account for this variation.

Reference range data are not available from our laboratories due to the low numbers of this species used.

The following pictures are stained with modified Wright's stain unless otherwise stated.

Atlas of Comparative Diagnostic and Experimental Hematology, Second Edition. Clifford Smith, Alfred Jarecki.
© 2011 Blackwell Publishing Ltd. Published 2011 by Blackwell Publishing Ltd.

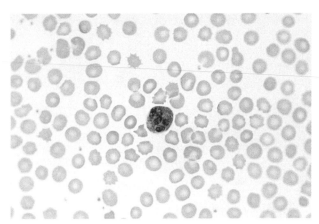

Photo 2.1 Rabbit: peripheral blood. Normal neutrophil, superficially resembling eosinophils but containing smaller, punctate, pink granules. Neutrophil lobulation is also more developed (×1000).

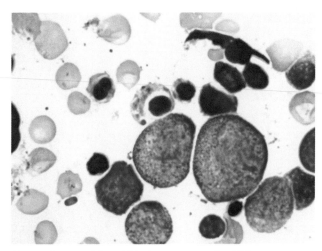

Photo 2.4 Healthy rabbit: bone marrow (×1000).

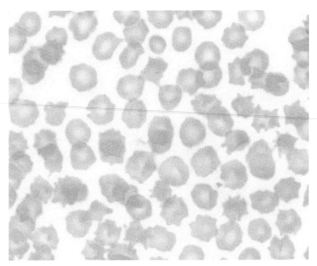

Photo 2.2 Healthy rabbit: peripheral blood. "Thorn apple" red cells (×1000).

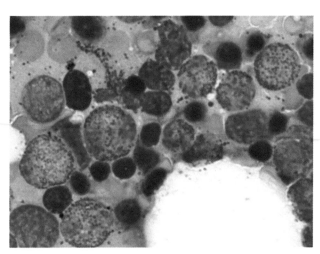

Photo 2.5 Healthy rabbit: bone marrow (×1000).

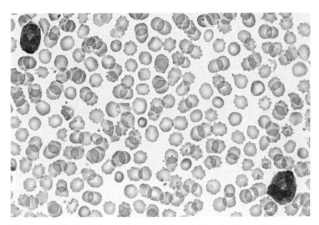

Photo 2.3 Healthy rabbit: peripheral blood. Basophils, "thorn apple" red cells and anisocytosis (×1000).

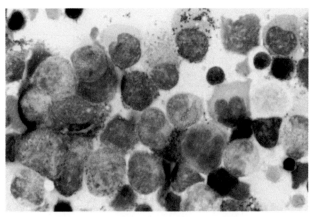

Photo 2.6 Healthy rabbit: bone marrow (×1000).

References

1. Marco I, Cuenca R, Pastor J, Velarde R, Lavin S (2003). Hematology and serum chemistry values of the European brown hare. *Vet Clin Pathol* 32(4): 195–198.
2. Feldman BF, Zinkl JG, Jain NC (eds) (2010). *Schalm's Veterinary Hematology (6th edn)*. Baltimore: Lippincott Williams & Wilkins.
3. Kabata J, Gratwohl A, Tichelli A, John L, Speck B (1991). Haematologic values of New Zealand white rabbits determined by automated flow cytometry. *Lab Anim Sci* 41: 613–619.
4. Harkness JE, Wagner JE (1995). *The Biology and Medicine of Rabbits and Rodents (4th edn)*. Baltimore: Williams and Wilkins.
5. Johnson-Delaney CA (1996). *Exotic Companion Medicine Handbook*. Lake Worth: Wingers Publishing.
6. Hillyer EV, Quesenberry KE (1997). *Ferrets, Rabbits and Rodents – Clinical Medicine and Surgery*. Philadelphia: WB Saunders.

3

Cat

Introduction

Cats are most likely encountered in veterinary medicine. Rarely used in toxicological studies, they are not good predictors of treatment-related findings in man and difficult to keep in a controlled environment, complicating already variable "normal/reference/background" values.

Feral animals will exhibit much wider ranges of values than domesticated animals which in any case are very breed dependent[1].

Blood picture

Red cell counts are higher in male animals than in females, with mean corpuscular volume (MCV) values approximately half those of humans[2]. Blood smears often exhibit rouleaux and moderate anisocytosis, and Heinz bodies are usual in normal healthy animals. Reticulocytes exhibit an aggregate or punctuate appearance.

White cells and differential counts are more variable than those of dogs especially in apprehensive animals. The majority leukocyte is the neutrophil which may contain Döhle bodies[3], and have prominent Barr bodies (nuclear drumstick appendages).

Platelet counts are more variable than is observed in the dog and human, with similar morphology, although clumping may be problematic[4].

Reference range data are not available from our laboratories.

The following pictures are stained with modified Wright's stain unless otherwise stated.

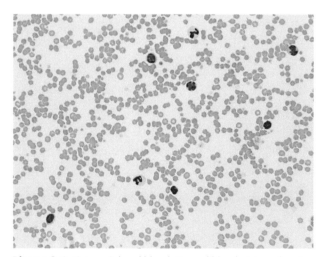

Photo 3.1 Cat: peripheral blood. Normal blood picture showing neutrophils and lymphocytes (×500).

Atlas of Comparative Diagnostic and Experimental Hematology, Second Edition. Clifford Smith, Alfred Jarecki.
© 2011 Blackwell Publishing Ltd. Published 2011 by Blackwell Publishing Ltd.

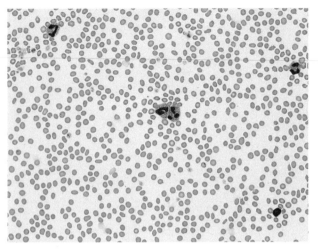

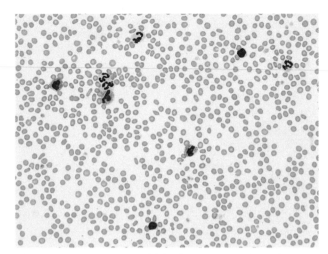

Photo 3.2 Cat: peripheral blood. Blood picture with unexplained eosinophilia; lymphocytes are small with little cytoplasm (×500).

Photo 3.3 Cat: peripheral blood. Same animal as Photo 3.2 (×500).

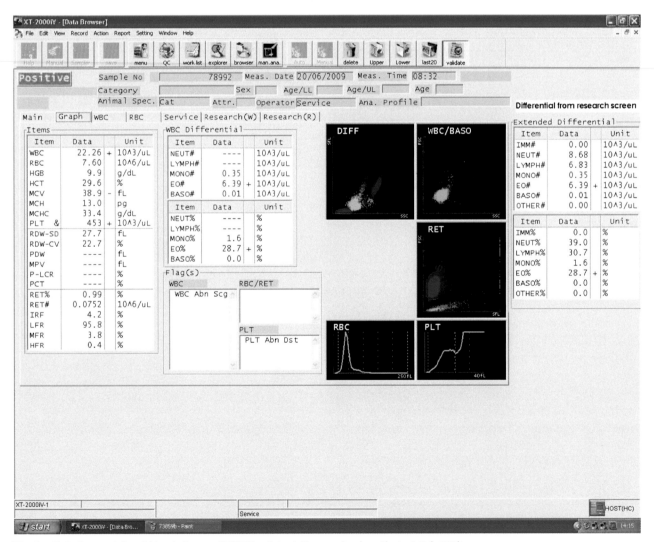

Photo 3.4 Cat: peripheral blood. Sysmex XT2000 printout. Same animal as Photo 3.2 (×500).

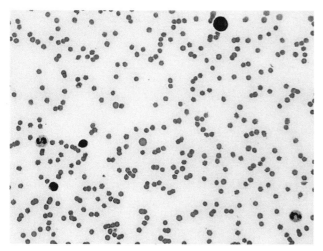

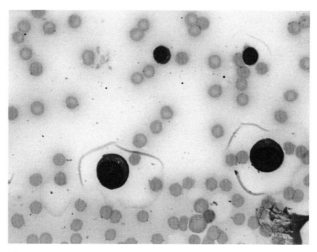

Photo 3.5 Cat: peripheral blood. Sudden onset of anemia and collapse. Severe anemia combined with a very low platelet count (×500).

Photo 3.6 Cat: peripheral blood. Same animal as Photo 3.5. Undifferentiated mononuclear cells that are large with round to oval eccentrically placed nuclei, coarse granular chromatin and moderate amounts of deep blue cytoplasm. Intermediate and late normoblasts are present. Cells are surrounded by a ring of protein (×500).

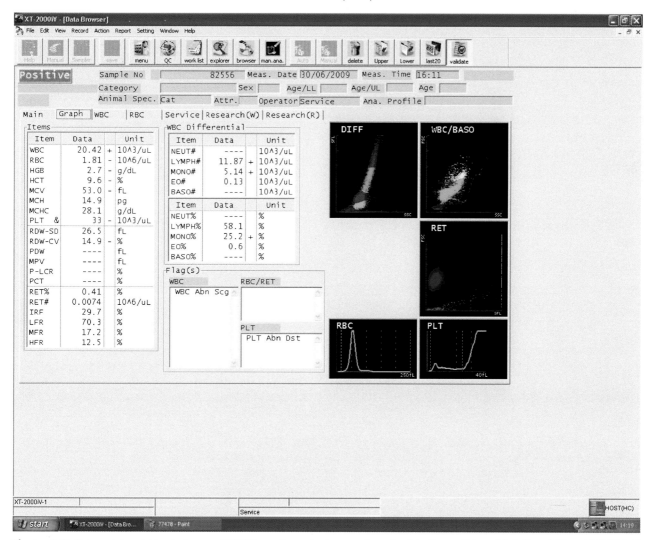

Photo 3.7 Cat: peripheral blood. Sysmex XT2000 results and cytogram for animal in Photos 3.5 and 3.6. Note Diff and WBC/BASO cytograms.

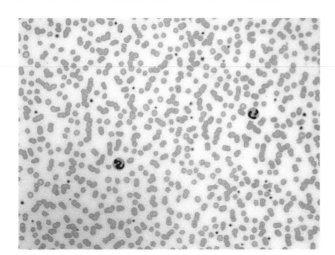

Photo 3.8 Cat: peripheral blood. Rouleaux (×500).

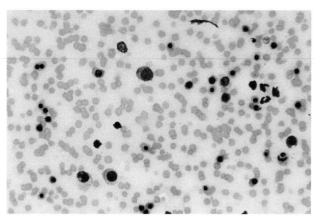

Photo 3.11 Cat: peripheral blood. Feline leukemia virus. Erythroleukemia; nucleated red cells and lymphocytes (×500).

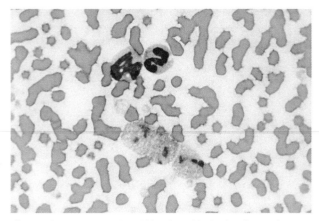

Photo 3.9 Cat: peripheral blood. Döhle bodies (×1000).

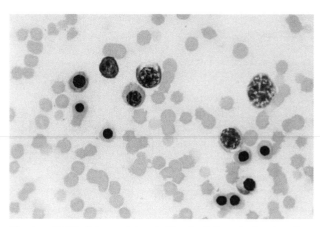

Photo 3.12 Cat: peripheral blood. Feline leukemia virus. Erythroleukemia; nucleated red cells and atypical lymphocytes (×1000).

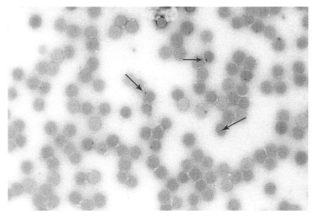

Photo 3.10 Cat: peripheral blood. Heinz bodies stained with methyl blue (arrowed) (×1000).

References

1. O'Brien M, Murphy MG, Lowe JA (1998). Haematology and clinical chemistry parameters in the cat (*Felis domesticus*). *J Nutr* 128: 2678S–2679S.
2. Feldman BF, Zinkl JG, Jain NC (eds) (2010). *Schalm's Veterinary Hematology (6th edn)*. Baltimore: Lippincott Williams & Wilkins.
3. Kahn CM (2005). *The Merck Veterinary Manual (10th edn)*. Philadelphia: National Publishing Inc.
4. Meyer DJ, Harvey JW (2005). *Veterinary Laboratory Medicine: Interpretation and Diagnosis (3rd edn)*. St. Louis: WB Saunders.

4

Dog

Introduction

Beagles are a popular choice of pet in addition to probably being the most widely encountered large animal experimental breed. Reference values reflect the specific population of animals, being tighter for experimental animals than those presenting at veterinary clinics.

Blood picture

A diurnal rhythm has been reported in beagle red cell, hematocrit and hemoglobin values, being highest in the early morning, declining throughout the day and increasing in the evening. These changes, due to splenic contraction, are also seen following feeding and notably following exercise and stress. Breeds bred for racing, especially the Greyhound, show this effect much more markedly.

Strain variation in mean corpuscular volume (MCV) is large; Jain[1] cites a range of MCVs from less than 55 fL (in the Japanese Akita and Shiba dogs) to greater than 106 fL (in some Toy and Miniature Poodles). Anisocytosis is therefore usual; erythrocyte diameters ranging from 5.5–7.5 μM and RDWs of 11.5–16.0% are common.

The mean cell hemoglobin concentration (MCHC) in all but very young animals (where it is reduced) is constant at around 33.1 g/dL.

Normally, few polychromatic cells are present in the adult dog. Reticulocytes are released from the bone marrow in an oscillatory manner approximately every 14 days[1], with a variable release rate and intravascular maturation time.

Occasional nucleated red cells and infrequent Howell–Jolly bodies may be seen on the blood smear and are quite normal in healthy animals.

Diurnal and seasonal rhythms may also be seen in leukocytes (principally neutrophils), although these changes are small. Conditioned animals will have lower leukocyte counts than animals newly arrived in kennels[1], and transient stress-related increases may also be observed.

Blood films from healthy animals usually show a reactive neutrophilia – inverse neutrophil : lymphocyte ratios are not uncommon. The distribution of nuclear lobulation in canine neutrophils is slightly left-shifted in comparison with human cells[2]. Granulation in the mature neutrophil is relatively indistinct and may appear absent in Romanowsky films. It is notable that alkaline phosphatase is difficult or even impossible to demonstrate by conventional cytochemical techniques whereas this lack of staining is not paralleled by peroxidase or chloroacetate esterase.

Lymphocytes are generally readily identifiable and a proportion may appear "atypical" or "reactive"; they may contain red to azurophilic cytoplasmic granules.

Monocytes may be confused with juvenile neutrophils as nuclei shapes are extremely variable; they may be round, multi-lobulated, band-shaped, or S-shaped. The cytoplasm may contain vacuoles and faint azurophilic granules.

Atlas of Comparative Diagnostic and Experimental Hematology, Second Edition. Clifford Smith, Alfred Jarecki.
© 2011 Blackwell Publishing Ltd. Published 2011 by Blackwell Publishing Ltd.

Canine eosinophil nuclei usually only have two or three lobes. Eosinophils are clearly identifiable, although their granules are extremely variable in number and size. Their cytoplasm is basophilic, and may contain vacuoles. Adult greyhound eosinophils commonly lack distinct granules and contain clear vacuoles, although the granules of pups are a dark gray colour.

Canine basophils, rarely seen in blood films, possess a scattering of large basophilic granules.

Canine platelets are present in similar numbers, and are similar in size and shape to those of man, but exhibit anisocytosis.

Typical ranges (Siemens Advia 120)

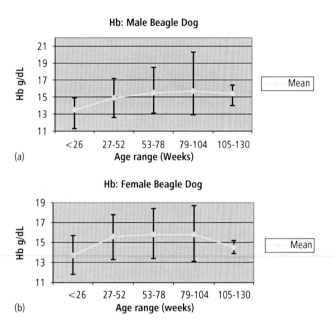

Figure 4.1 Beagle: hemoglobin (Hb). Male (a) and female (b) animals.

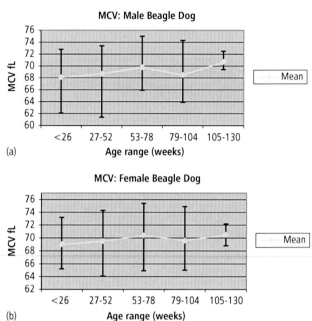

Figure 4.3 Beagle: mean cell volume (MCV). Male (a) and female (b) animals.

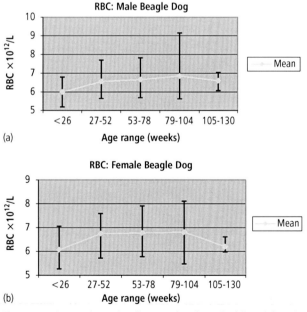

Figure 4.2 Beagle: red cell count (RBC). Male (a) and female (b) animals.

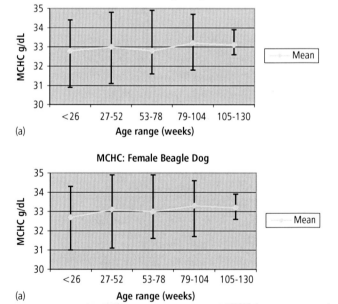

Figure 4.4 Beagle: mean cell hemoglobin concentration (MCHC). Male (a) and female (b) animals.

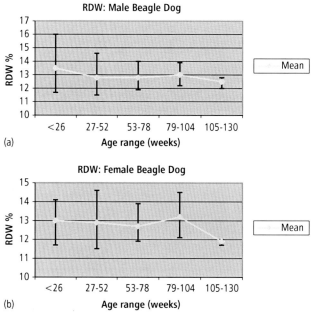

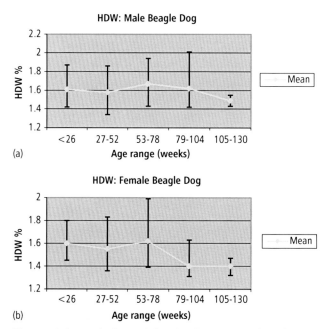

Figure 4.5 Beagle: red cell distribution width (RDW). Male (a) and female (b) animals.

Figure 4.6 Beagle: hemoglobin distribution width (HDW). Male (a) and female (b) animals.

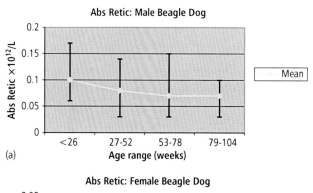

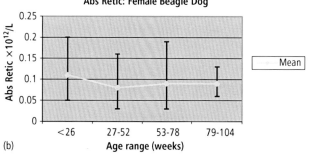

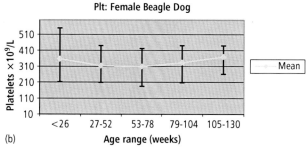

Figure 4.7 Beagle: absolute reticulocyte count (Retic Abs). Male (a) and female (b) animals.

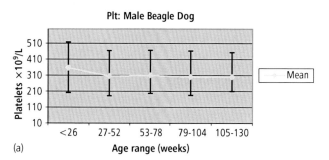

Figure 4.8 Beagle: platelet count (PLT). Male (a) and female (b) animals.

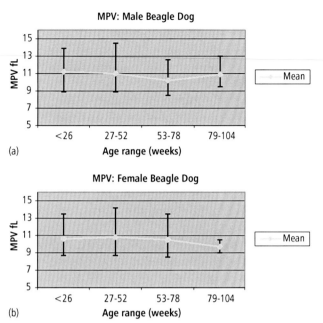

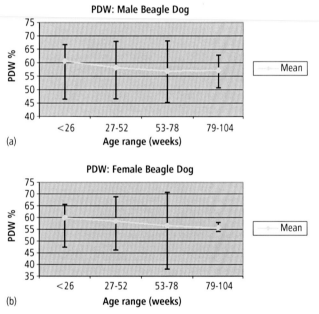

Figure 4.9 Beagle: mean platelet volume (MPV). Male (a) and female (b) animals.

Figure 4.10 Beagle: platelet distribution width (PDW). Male (a) and female (b) animals.

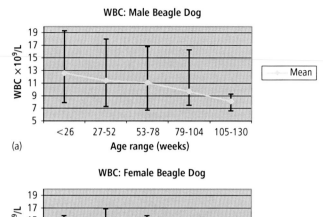

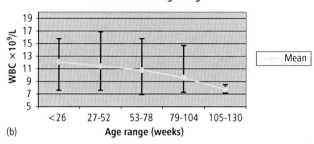

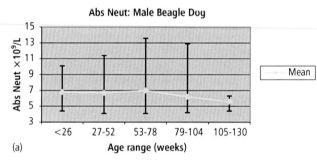

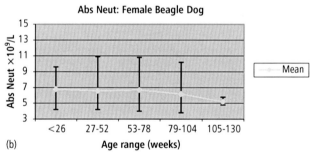

Figure 4.11 Beagle: total white cell count (WBC). Male (a) and female (b) animals.

Figure 4.12 Beagle: neutrophil count (Neut). Male (a) and female (b) animals.

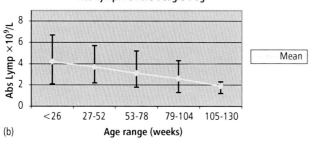

(a)

(b)

Figure 4.13 Beagle: lymphocyte count (Lymph). Male (a) and female (b) animals.

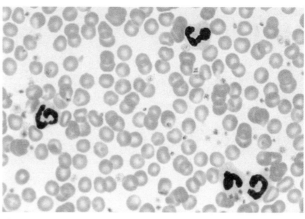

Photo 4.2 Beagle: peripheral blood. Normal blood picture (×1000).

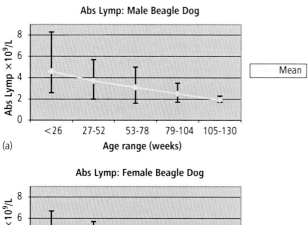

Photo 4.1 Beagle: peripheral blood. Normal blood picture showing neutrophils (×500).

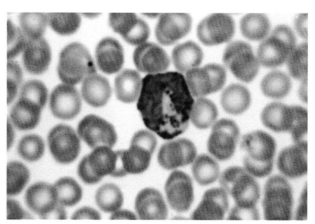

Photo 4.3 Beagle: peripheral blood. Normal blood picture, basophil (×1000).

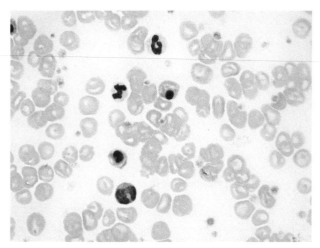

Photo 4.4 Beagle: peripheral blood. Nucleated red cells and moderate polychromasia (×1000).

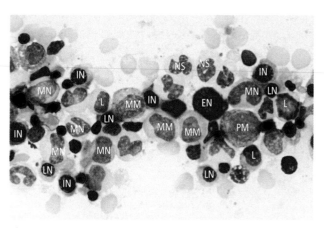

Photo 4.7 Beagle: bone marrow. Key: EN, early normoblast; IN, intermediate normoblast; LN, late normoblast; PM, promyelocyte; MM, myelocyte; MN metamyelocyte; L, lymphocyte (×1000).

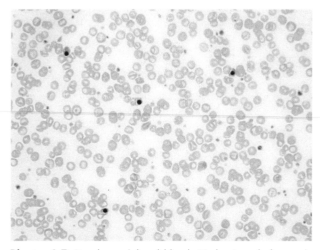

Photo 4.5 Beagle: peripheral blood. Moderate polychromasia and nucleated red cells. Some red cells are suspiciously like target cells. Same animal as Photo 4.4 (×500).

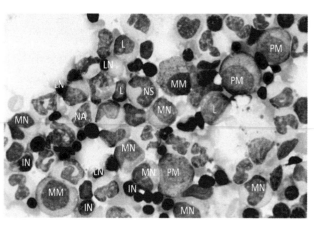

Photo 4.8 Beagle: bone marrow. Key: EN, early normoblast; IN, intermediate normoblast; LN, late normoblast; PM, promyelocyte; MM, myelocyte; MN metamyelocyte; L, lymphocyte (×1000).

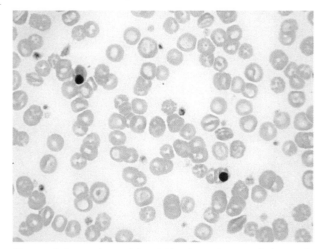

Photo 4.6 Beagle: peripheral blood. Moderate polychromasia and nucleated red cells. Same animal as Photo 4.4 (×1000).

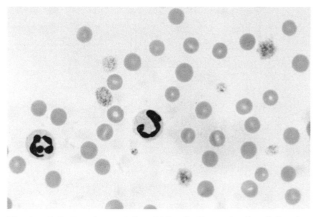

Photo 4.9 Beagle: peripheral blood. Giant platelets following gastrointestinal bleed (×1000).

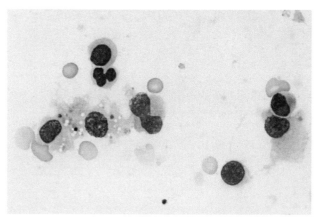

Photo 4.10 Beagle: peripheral blood. Aplastic anemia showing macrophages (×1000).

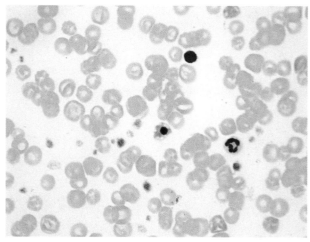

Photo 4.13 Beagle: peripheral blood. Polychromasia and nucleated red cells (×1000).

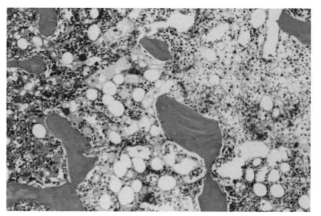

Photo 4.11 Beagle: bone marrow section. Hypoplasia. H&E stain (×40).

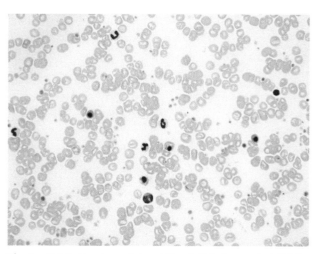

Photo 4.14 Beagle: peripheral blood. Polychromasia (×500).

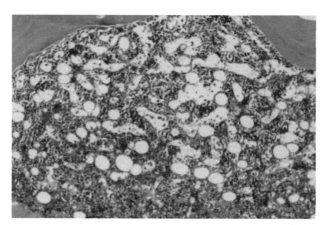

Photo 4.12 Beagle: bone marrow section. Hypoplasia. H&E stain (×40).

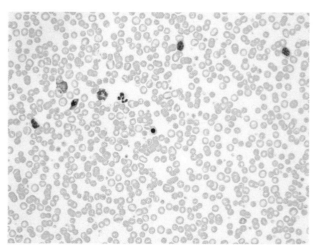

Photo 4.15 Beagle: peripheral blood. Polychromasia, nucleated red cells and vacuolated monocyte (×500).

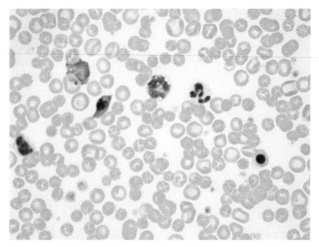

Photo 4.16 Beagle: peripheral blood. Polychromasia, nucleated red cells and vacuolated monocyte (×1000).

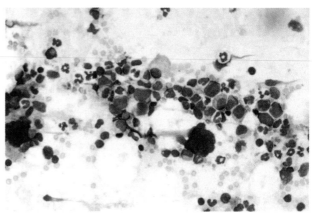

Photo 4.18 Beagle: bone marrow. Erythroid hypoplasia (×500).

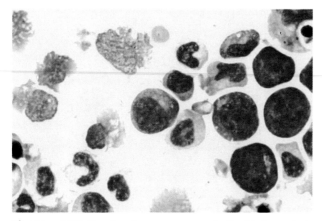

Photo 4.17 Beagle: bone marrow. Erythroid hypoplasia (×1000).

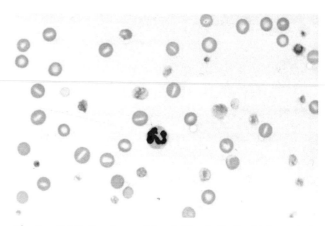

Photo 4.19 Beagle: peripheral blood. Erythroid hypoplasia (×200).

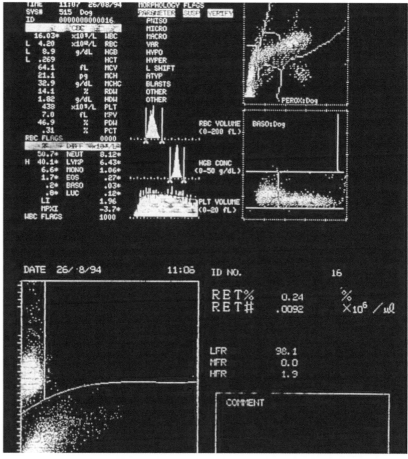

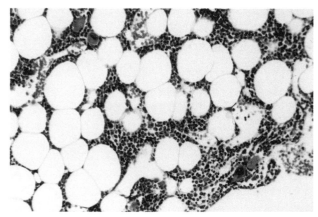

Photo 4.20 Beagle: peripheral blood. Erythroid hypoplasia. Technicon H1 printout. Same animal as Photo 4.19.

Photo 4.21 Beagle: bone marrow section. Hypoplastic spaces (×400).

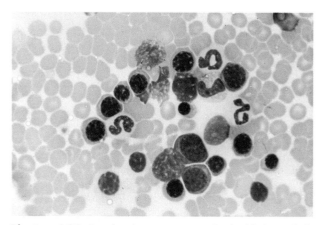

Photo 4.22 Beagle: bone marrow. Erythroid hypoplasia (×1000).

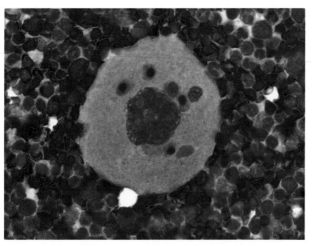

Photo 4.23 Beagle: bone marrow. Emperipolesis in a megakaryocyte (×1000).

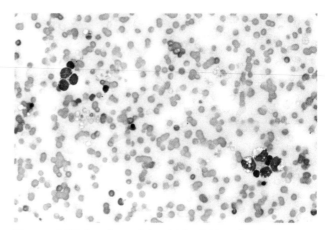

Photo 4.26 Beagle: peripheral blood. Vacuolated monocytes (×500).

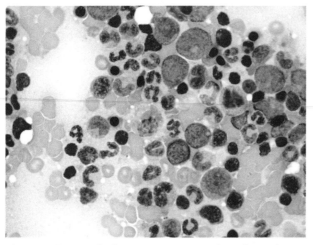

Photo 4.24 Beagle: bone marrow. Macrophage (×1000).

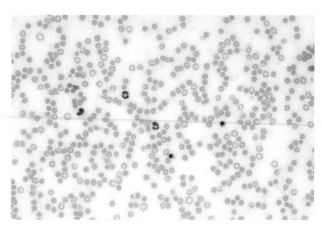

Photo 4.27 Beagle: peripheral blood. Autoimmune hemolytic anemia (×500).

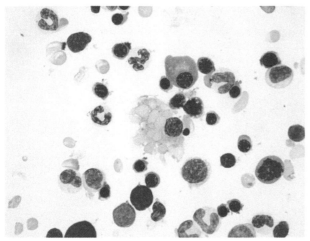

Photo 4.25 Beagle: bone marrow. Erythrophagocytosis (×1000).

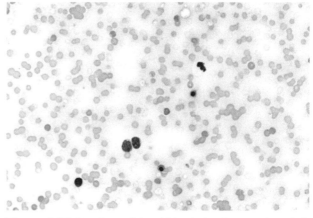

Photo 4.28 Beagle: peripheral blood. Autoimmune hemolytic anemia (×500).

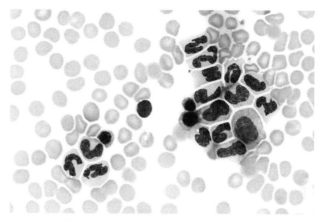

Photo 4.29 Beagle: bone marrow. Recovery from agranulocytosis (×1000).

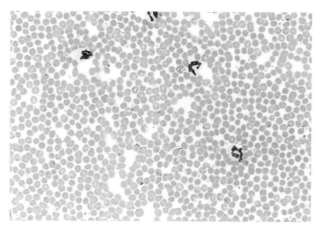

Photo 4.32 Beagle: peripheral blood. Bacteremia (×500).

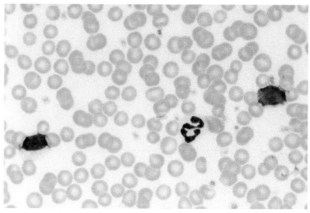

Photo 4.30 Beagle: peripheral blood. Atypical lymphocytes (×1000).

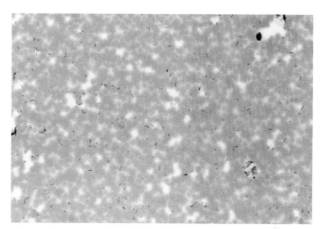

Photo 4.33 Beagle: peripheral blood. Bacteremia (×500).

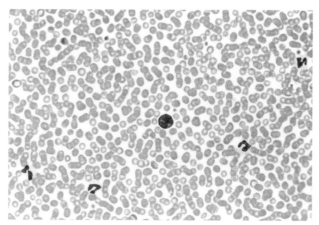

Photo 4.31 Beagle: peripheral blood. Atypical lymphocyte (×500).

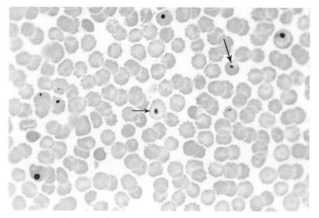

Photo 4.34 Beagle: peripheral blood. Distemper bodies (arrowed); uncommonly seen in this condition, these viral inclusions resemble Howell–Jolly bodies (×1000).

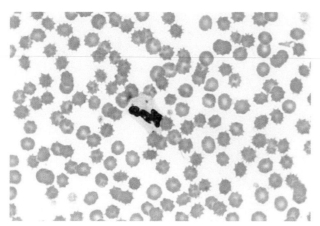

Photo 4.35 Beagle: peripheral blood. Döhle bodies (aggregates of rough endoplasmic reticulum) (×1000).

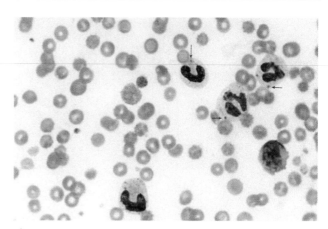

Photo 4.36 Beagle: peripheral blood. Döhle bodies with giant platelets (normal in dogs) (×1000).

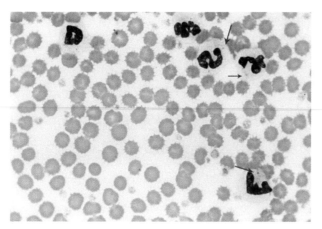

Photo 4.37 Beagle: peripheral blood. Döhle bodies (arrowed), less obvious in this animal (×1000).

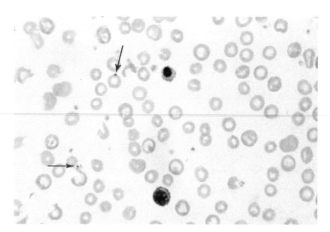

Photo 4.38 Beagle: peripheral blood. Heinz body-positive anemia with nucleated red cells (arrowed) (×1000).

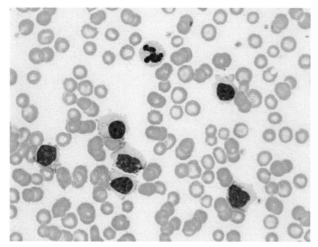

Photo 4.39 Poodle: peripheral blood. Lymphoma: the majority of lymphocytes are large with abundant cytoplasm (×1000).

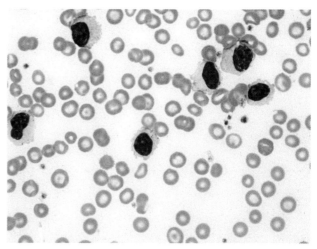

Photo 4.40 Poodle: peripheral blood. Lymphoma: same animal as Photo 4.39 (×1000).

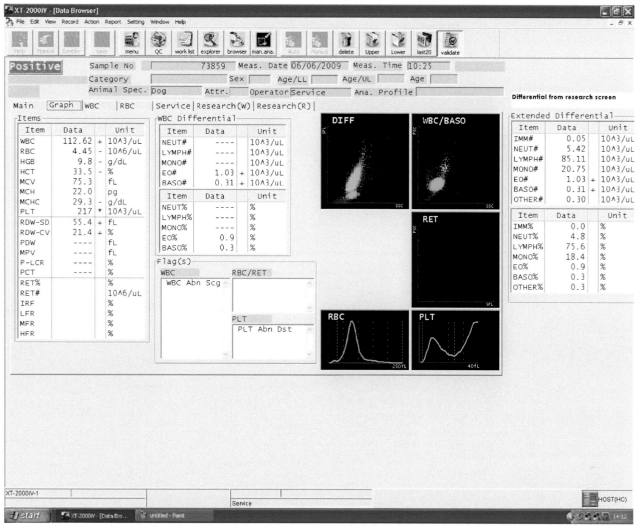

Photo 4.41 Poodle: peripheral blood. Sysmex XT2000 printout. Lymphoma: same animal as Photo 4.39.

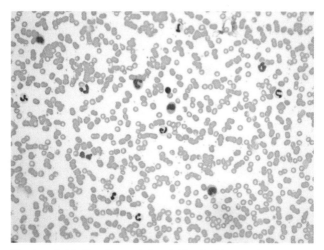

Photo 4.42 Beagle: peripheral blood. Abnormal monocytes and neutrophilia with a left shift (×500).

CBC			
WBC:	H	37.88	x10³ cells/ μL
RBC:	L	5.00	x10⁶ cells/ μL
HGB:	L	12.3	g/dL
HCT:	L	34.4	%
MCV:		68.2	fL
MCH:		24.1	pg
MCHC:		35.1	g/dL
CHCM:		35.5	g/dL
CH:		24.3	pg
CHDW:		3.03	pg
RDW:		13.3	%
HDW:		1.35	g/dL
PLT:	H	777	x10³ cells/ μL
MPV:		3.3	fL
PDW:	H	31.4	%
PCT:	L	0.60	%

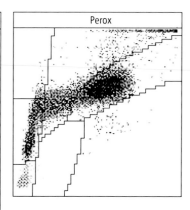

Perox

WBC Differential			
		%	x10³ cells/ μL
WBC:		H	37.88
Neut:	H	78.7	29.83
Lymph:	L	9.5	3.59
Mono:		11.0	4.18
Eos:		0.3	0.10
Baso:		0.1	0.06
LUC:		0.4	0.14
LI:			2.88
MPXI:			20.7

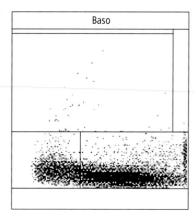

Baso

Photo 4.43 Beagle: peripheral blood. Advia 120 printout. Same animal as Photo 4.42.

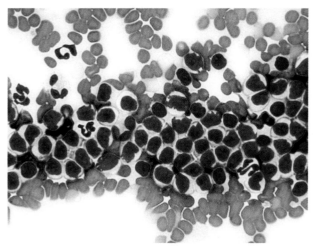

Photo 4.44 Beagle: peripheral blood. Lymphoma (×1000).

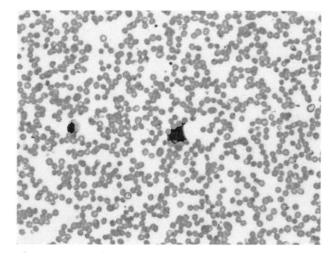

Photo 4.45 Labrador: peripheral blood. Four-year-old male animal diagnosed with lymphoma showing atypical lymphocytes (×500).

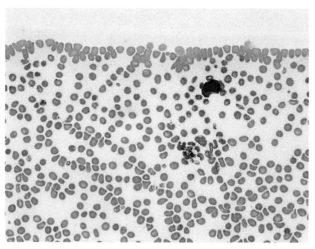

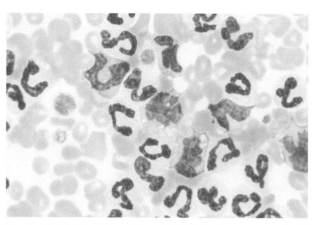

Photo 4.48 Spaniel: peripheral blood. Toxic monocytes. MGG (×1000).

Photo 4.46 Labrador: peripheral blood. Same animal as Photo 4.45 demonstrating atypical lymphocytes (×500).

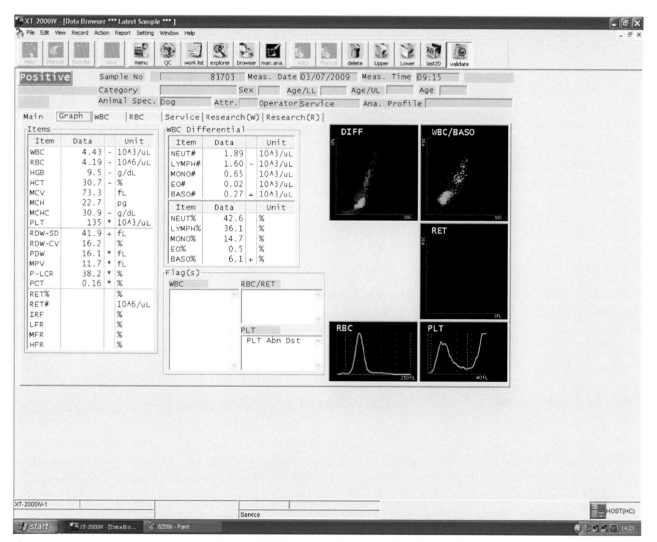

Photo 4.47 Labrador: peripheral blood. Sysmex XT2000 printout. Same animal as Photo 4.45.

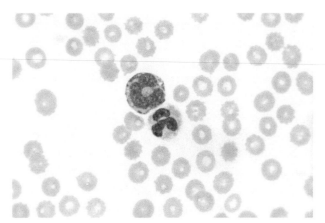

Photo 4.49 Spaniel: peripheral blood. Toxic monocyte. MGG (×1000).

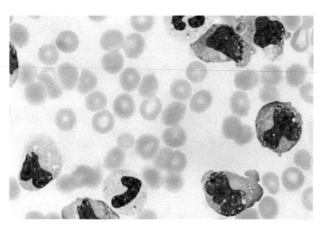

Photo 4.52 Spaniel: peripheral blood. Toxic monocytes with non-segmented neutrophils (×1000).

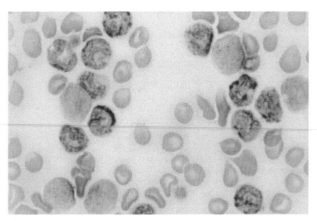

Photo 4.50 Spaniel: peripheral blood. Toxic monocytes. Dual esterase (×1000).

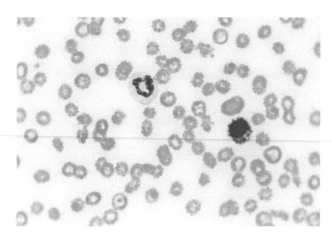

Photo 4.53 Dog: peripheral blood. Circulating mast cell (×500).

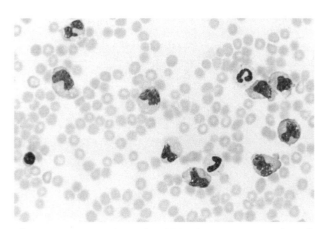

Photo 4.51 Spaniel: peripheral blood. Toxic monocytes (×500).

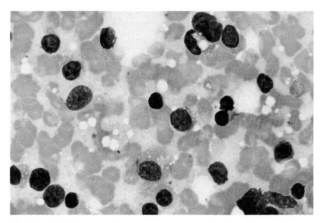

Photo 4.54 Dog: bone marrow. Aplastic picture. Foamy macrophages in thick part of the smear. (×1000).

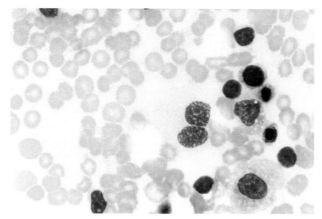

Photo 4.55 Dog: bone marrow. Aplastic picture. Foamy macrophages: same animal as Photo 4.54. (×100).

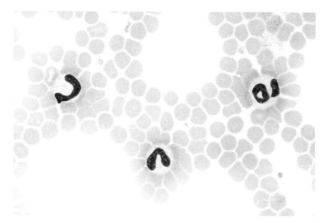

Photo 4.58 Dog: peripheral blood. Pseudo Pelger–Huët neutrophils; occasional cells were observed with normal lobulation (×1000).

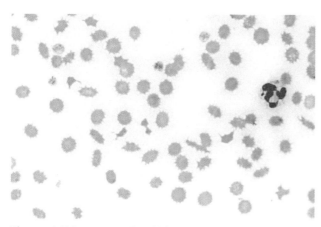

Photo 4.56 Dog: peripheral blood. Uremia; large numbers of Burr cells present (×1000).

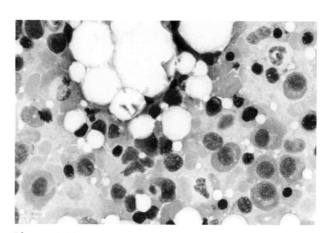

Photo 4.59 Dog: bone marrow. Myeloma (×1000).

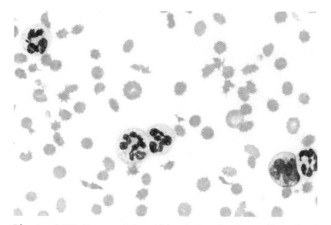

Photo 4.57 Dog: peripheral blood. Uremia; Burr cells and red cell fragments (×1000).

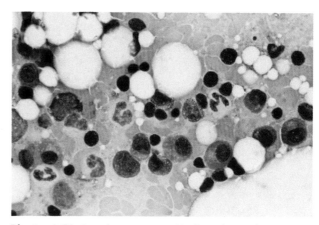

Photo 4.60 Dog: bone marrow. Myeloma (×1000).

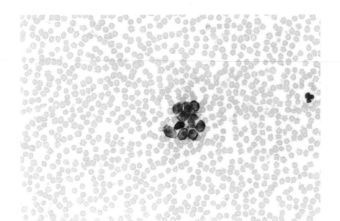

Photo 4.61 Dog: peripheral blood. Lymphocyte aggregates (×500).

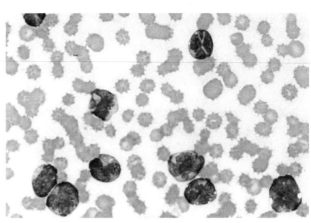

Photo 4.64 Dog: peripheral blood. Lymphoma with cleft nuclei (×1000).

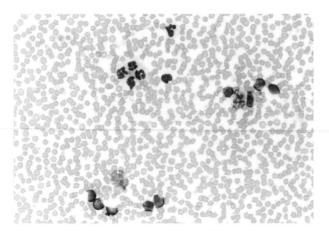

Photo 4.62 Dog: peripheral blood. White cell aggregates (×500).

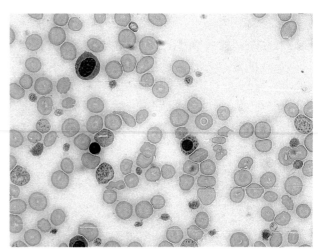

Photo 4.65 Dog: peripheral blood. Post treatment with a novel anti-malarial compound; nucleated red cells and basophilic stippling (×1000).

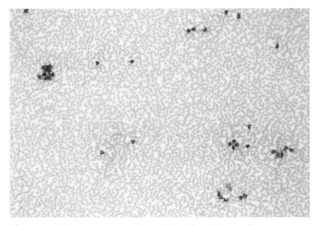

Photo 4.63 Dog: peripheral blood. White cell aggregates (×400).

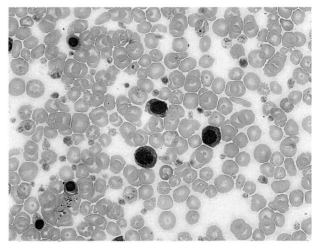

Photo 4.66 Dog: peripheral blood. Same animal as Photo 4.65, with nucleated red cells and basophilic stippling (×1000).

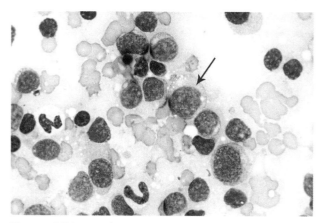

Photo 4.70 Dog: bone marrow. Lymphoma. The majority of cells present are infiltrating malignant cells (arrowed) sample obtained at autopsy (×1000).

Photo 4.67 Dog: bone marrow. Same animal as Photo 4.65 with marked erythroid hyperplasia (×1000).

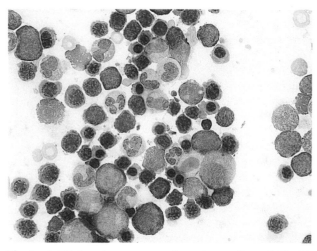

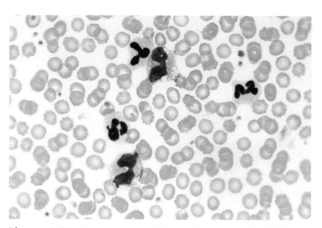

Photo 4.71 Dog: peripheral blood. Monocytosis (×1000).

Photo 4.68 Dog: bone marrow. Same dog as Photo 4.65 with marked erythroid hyperplasia (×1000).

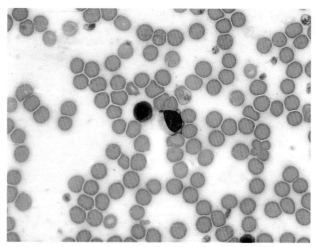

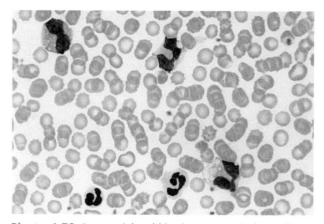

Photo 4.72 Dog: peripheral blood. Monocytosis (×1000).

Photo 4.69 Dog: peripheral blood. The difference and similarity between a lymphocyte and nucleated red cell (×1000).

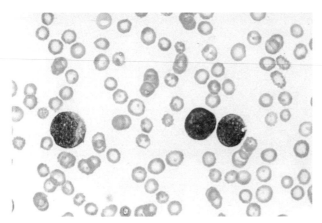

Photo 4.73 Bloodhound: peripheral blood. Lymphoma with chronic anemia exhibiting hypochromia (×1000).

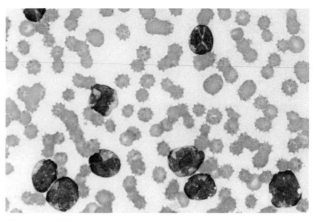

Photo 4.76 Beagle: peripheral blood. Severe crenation and lymphoblasts in an animal with renal failure associated with lymphoma (×1000).

References

1. Feldman BF, Zinkl JG, Jain NC (eds) (2010). *Schalm's Veterinary Hematology (6th edn)*. Baltimore: Lippincott Williams & Wilkins.
2. Kennedy WP, Climenko DR (1931). Studies on the Arneth Count – XVIII. The normal count in various mammals. *Exp Physiol* 21(3): 253–264.

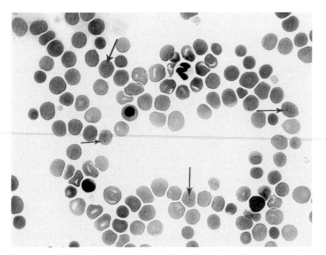

Photo 4.74 Dog: peripheral blood. Red cell regeneration showing nucleated red cells and possible inclusion bodies (arrowed) (×500).

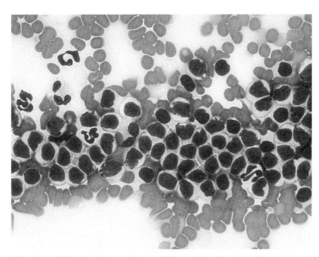

Photo 4.75 Jack Russell: peripheral blood. Lymphoid aggregates in lymphocytic leukemia (×500).

5

Monkey

Introduction

Old world primates encountered in comparative hematology most often emanate from commercial breeding sources unless they are from zoological sources or are required for specific age-related testing in preclinical studies; wild-captured stock are rare and generally avoided for preclinical studies due to the wide variation in values for most parameters due to factors such as health status, age, geographic origin, etc.

New world primates such as the marmoset are also readily available from commercial breeding sources with many centers having established their own breeding colonies. Samples from rhesus and chimpanzee are rarely received in the laboratory as use of these species in research has diminished due to animal welfare concerns: it is now very rare for preclinical laboratories to receive samples from these species for routine analysis.

Blood picture

Erythrocyte counts and hemoglobin values in male animals are marginally higher than in females with mean corpuscular volume (MCV) ranging from less than 40 fL to greater than 150 fL, often with a lower mean cell hemoglobin concentration (MCHC) than in human samples (typically 26–29 g/dL). Erythrocyte diameter in macaques measures around 6.4–7.7 μm[1,2].

Few polychromatic cells are present in healthy individuals, with reticulocyte counts of <2.0% being common. Anisocytosis may be encountered in squirrel monkeys, with Howell–Jolly bodies and occasional punctuate basophilia.

Total white cell counts are often higher in healthy female animals than in males. The neutrophil nucleus may have up to 12 lobes[3], and the granules of the cytoplasm are pink and closely packed. Up to 2% band forms is normal.

Neutrophil:lymphocyte ratios can vary greatly meaning greater emphasis must be placed on absolute values for data interpretation.

Lymphocytes resemble their human counterparts, although "atypical" or "reactive" cells (i.e. cells with abundant and/or intensely basophilic cytoplasm) may commonly be seen. Lymphocytes of squirrel monkeys are fragile and break up on preparation of a blood smear, appearing microscopically as "smear" cells.

Monocytes also resemble those in humans, although vacuolated cells may be more common; they may sometimes be easily confused with juvenile neutrophils.

Eosinophils are easily identifiable, as they are very similar to those of humans, although they are often present in greater numbers than observed in humans; values of around 8% are unremarkable. The nucleus is generally non-segmented or bi-lobed.

Basophil granules tend to be relatively few in number, may vary considerably in diameter and do

Atlas of Comparative Diagnostic and Experimental Hematology, Second Edition. Clifford Smith, Alfred Jarecki.
© 2011 Blackwell Publishing Ltd. Published 2011 by Blackwell Publishing Ltd.

not normally obscure the nucleus. Basophils are comparatively common with values of 3% being unexceptional.

Large unstained cells (LUCs) can constitute up to 5% of a normal population of circulating white blood cells, and reflect the same situation as in other species, i.e. increases are due to reactive, activated or atypical lymphocytes or mononuclear cells.

Platelet numbers are similar to those of humans with typical values of $150–400 \times 10^3/\mu L$, whilst mean platelet volume (MPV) and platelet distribution width (PDW) values are also similar.

MARMOSET

A wide range of hematological values is encountered in the marmoset due to the marked sensitivity of the marmoset to various stresses. A syndrome termed "wasting marmoset syndrome" (WMS)[4], manifests as

a Heinz body-positive hemolytic anemia, usually accompanied by muscle wasting, hair loss, failure to thrive, generalised weakness and often death. The appearance of a large number of Heinz bodies is a common finding in marmosets with WMS, although it is not diagnostic of the syndrome[5]. The addition of vitamin E and linoleic acid to the diet corrects *in vitro* hemolysis and affected marmosets show a remarkable improvement with lessening of the erythrocytic defect, probably as a result of correcting the phospholipid imbalance of the red cell membrane[6].

Anisocytosis, punctuate basophilia and stomatocytes may be observed in marmoset red cells.

Lymphocytes of marmosets are fragile and break up on preparation of a blood smear, appearing microscopically as "smear" cells.

Eosinophils, very similar to those of humans, are easily identifiable but the "muddy" gray–blue cytoplasm can make these cells less distinct.

Table 5.1 Typical ranges (Sysmex 4500) for group-housed and single-housed marmosets.

Group housed	Units	Male			Female		
		Mean	Min	Max	Mean	Min	Max
Hb	g/dL	10.2	7.2	12.3	9.7	6.3	11.9
RBC	$\times 10^6/\mu L$	7.28	5.20	9.01	7.28	4.45	8.83
MCV	fL	72.4	65.4	79.5	73.2	65.7	89.2
MCHC	g/dL	19.4	18.2	20.3	19.4	17.9	20.2
Retics	$\times 10^6/\mu L$	46.8	12.9	278.4	49.0	12.5	278.5
Plts	$\times 10^3/\mu L$	623	282	903	616	393	1018
WBC	$\times 10^3/\mu L$	6.1	2.4	14.6	6.0	1.8	13.9
Neuts (segmented)	%	53	23	81	50	17	80
Lymphs	%	42	10	74	46	15	81

Single housed	Units	Male			Female		
		Mean	Min	Max	Mean	Min	Max
Hb	g/dL	9.3	5.3	11.4	8.9	6.3	11.0
RBC	$\times 10^6/\mu L$	6.61	3.97	8.18	6.31	4.37	7.94
MCV	fL	72.5	61.3	83.0	73.1	62.9	84.2
MCHC	g/dL	19.5	16.8	20.7	19.4	17.4	20.8
Retics	$\times 10^6/\mu L$	78.3	14.3	585.0	93.3	15.8	371.0
Plts	$\times 10^3/\mu L$	590	133	1111	559	99	984
WBC	$\times 10^3/\mu L$	7.4	1.7	44.6	6.6	2.4	18.0
Neuts (segmented)	%	47	12	86	47	17	86
Lymphs	%	48	12	83	48	13	79

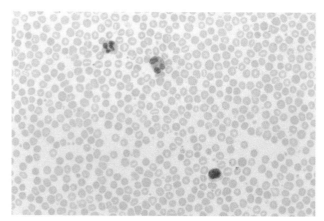

Photo 5.1 Marmoset: peripheral blood. Neutrophil, lymphocyte and eosinophil (×500).

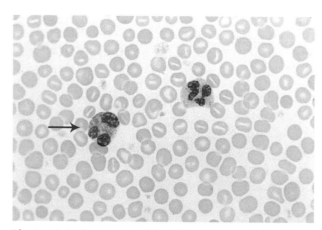

Photo 5.4 Marmoset: peripheral blood. Neutrophil and eosinophil (arrowed). Clarity of eosinophilic granules is not well marked but microscopic examination is relatively clear cut (×1000).

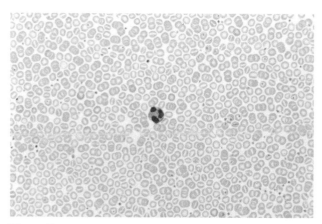

Photo 5.2 Marmoset: peripheral blood. Eosinophil and stomatocytes (×500).

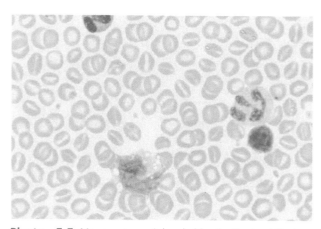

Photo 5.5 Marmoset: peripheral blood. Neutrophil, lymphocyte, vacuolated monocyte and eosinophil (×1000).

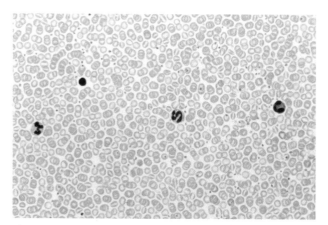

Photo 5.3 Marmoset: peripheral blood. Neutrophils and stomatocytes (×500).

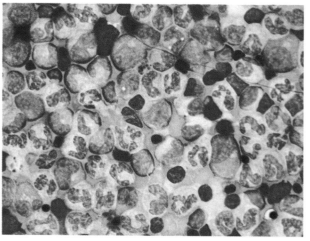

Photo 5.6 Marmoset: bone marrow (×1000).

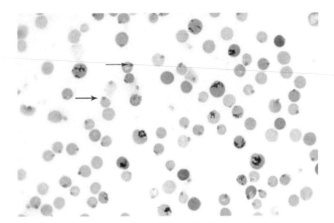

Photo 5.7 Marmoset: peripheral blood. New methylene blue (NMB) stain. A large number of Heinz bodies (arrowed) with a high reticulocyte count (×1000).

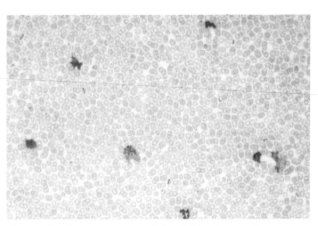

Photo 5.10 Marmoset: peripheral blood. Lymphocytes are fragile in this species, often producing smear cells (×500).

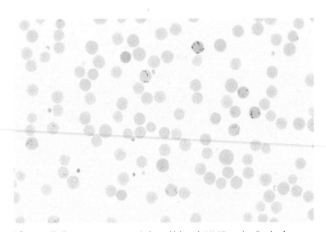

Photo 5.8 Marmoset: peripheral blood. NMB stain. Reticulocytes and Heinz bodies may be confused: compare and contrast with Photo 5.9 (×1000).

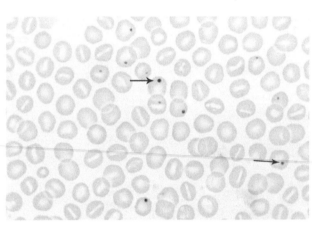

Photo 5.11 Marmoset: peripheral blood. Howell–Jolly bodies (arrowed) (×1000).

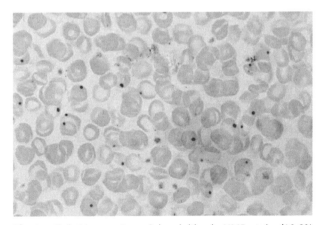

Photo 5.9 Marmoset: peripheral blood. NMB stain (10.8% Heinz bodies) (×1000).

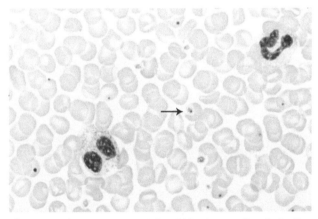

Photo 5.12 Marmoset: peripheral blood. Howell–Jolly bodies. Note the red cell overlaid with a platelet (arrowed) in contrast to the Howell–Jolly bodies (×1000).

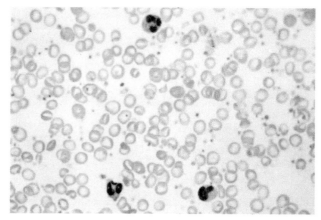

Photo 5.13 Marmoset: peripheral blood. Hypochromia and microcytosis; hemoglobin 5.6 g/dL (×500).

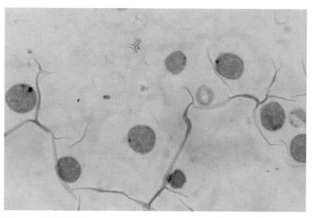

Photo 5.16 Marmoset: bone marrow. Lymphoma cells stained with ANAE (×1000).

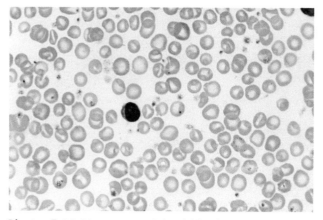

Photo 5.14 Marmoset: peripheral blood. Stomatocytes and basophilic stippling with Howell–Jolly bodies (×500).

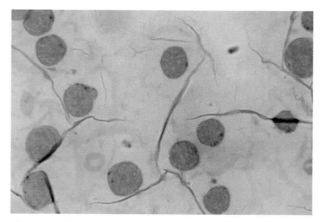

Photo 5.17 Marmoset: bone marrow. Lymphoma cells stained with ANAE (×1000).

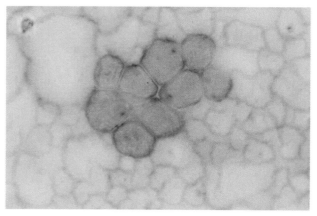

Photo 5.15 Marmoset: peripheral blood. Lymphoma cells stained with alpha naphthyl acetate esterase (ANAE) (×1000).

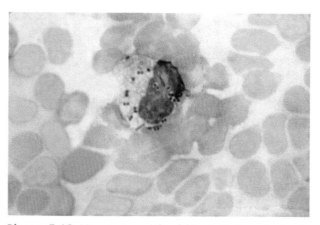

Photo 5.18 Marmoset: peripheral blood. Bacteremia due to infected in-dwelling arteriovenous shunt (×1000).

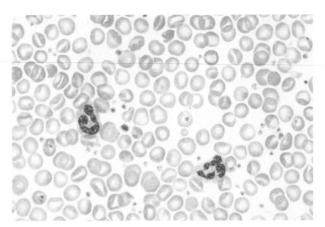

Photo 5.19 Marmoset: peripheral blood. Stomatocytes in a case of wasting marmoset syndrome (×1000).

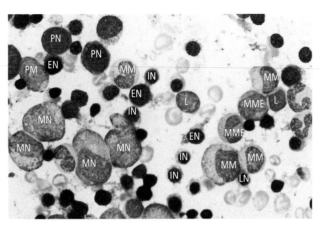

Photo 5.22 Marmoset: normal bone marrow. Key: EN, early normoblast; IN, intermediate normoblast; LN, late normoblast; MN, myelocyte neutrophil; MM, neutrophil metamyelocyte; MME, metamyelocyte eosinophil; L, lymphocyte (×1000).

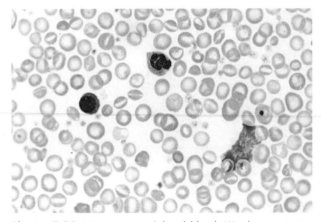

Photo 5.20 Marmoset: peripheral blood. Wasting marmoset syndrome. Hypochromia, stomatocytes, a normoblast and an occasional basophilic stippled cell are seen. Howell–Jolly bodies are a common finding in marmoset blood films (×1000).

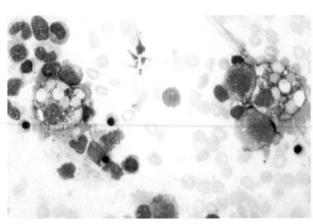

Photo 5.23 Marmoset: bone marrow. Two macrophages exhibiting erythrophagocytosis (×1000).

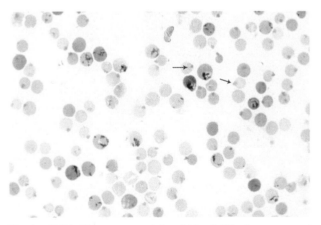

Photo 5.21 Marmoset: peripheral blood. Wasting marmoset syndrome. NMB stain for reticulocytes, additionally staining Heinz bodies (arrowed) (×1000).

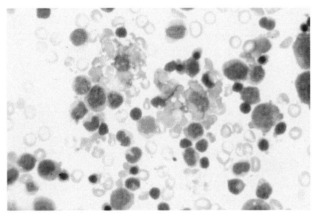

Photo 5.24 Marmoset: bone marrow. Erythrophagocytosis by macrophage (×1000).

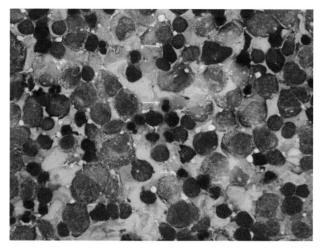

Photo 5.25 Marmoset: bone marrow. Multinucleate erythroblasts (×1000).

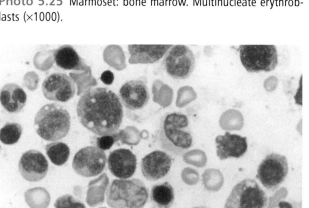

Photo 5.26 Marmoset: bone marrow. Vacuolation induced by ethanol termination (×1000).

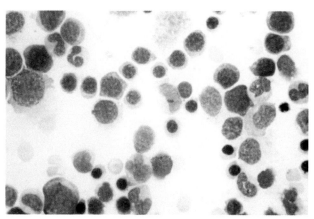

Photo 5.27 Marmoset: bone marrow. Erythroid hyperplasia (×1000).

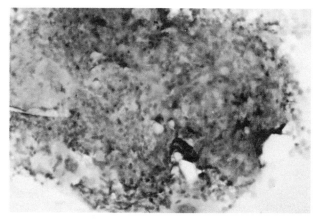

Photo 5.28 Marmoset: bone marrow. Perl's stain; low iron stores (×1000).

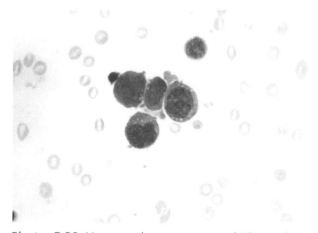

Photo 5.29 Marmoset: bone marrow. Myeloid vacuolation; artifact possibly due to barbiturate overdose (×1000).

CYNOMOLGUS

Introduction

Cynomolgus monkeys (old world primates) usually emanate from zoological sources or specialist breeders; wild-captured stock are extremely rare and generally avoided for preclinical studies due to the wide variation in values for most parameters due to factors such as health status, age, geographic origin etc.

Blood picture

Erythrocyte MCVs range approximately from 60–76 fL and there is usually a lower MCHC compared with other experimental animal species. Few polychromatic cells are normally present in healthy individuals, with reticulocyte counts variable, dependent on age and sex.

Total white cell counts in cynomolgus are extremely variable, emphasising the necessity to condition animals to blood collection and handling techniques, and to avoid the "panic reaction"[7].

Blood smears from healthy animals normally show a slight relative neutrophilia, but a wide variation from marked neutrophilia to marked relative lymphocytosis may occur. Neutrophil nuclear lobularity varies from comparative immaturity (band cells) to mature lobulation with occasional hyperlobulation (greater than five lobes). Granularity is generally slightly less distinct than in human cells.

Lymphocytes resemble their human counterparts although "atypical" or "reactive" cells are common.

Monocytes also resemble those of humans, although vacuolated cells may be more common, and confusion with juvenile neutrophils is possible.

Eosinophils are easily identifiable, as they are very similar to those of humans, and the nuclei are generally non-segmented or bi-lobed.

Basophils are comparatively common. The granules tend to be relatively few in number, vary considerably in diameter and do not normally obscure the nucleus.

Mean platelet diameter varies greatly, an observation which an inexperienced observer must not interpret as a hematological disorder.

Typical ranges (Siemens Advia 120)

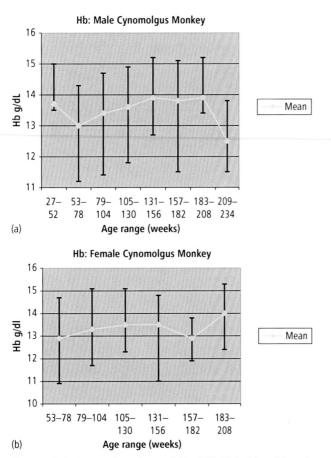

Figure 5.1 Cynomolgus: hemoglobin (Hb). Male (a) and female (b) animals.

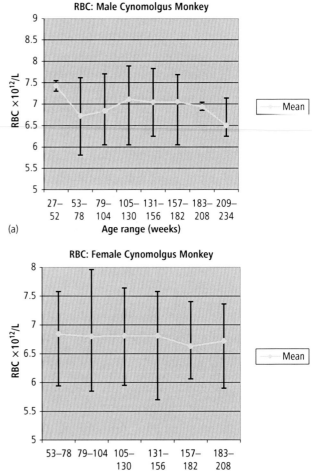

Figure 5.2 Cynomolgus: red cell count (RBC). Male (a) and female (b) animals.

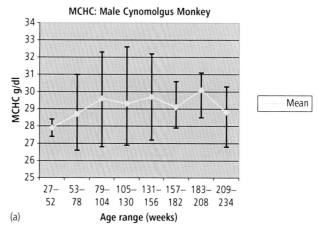

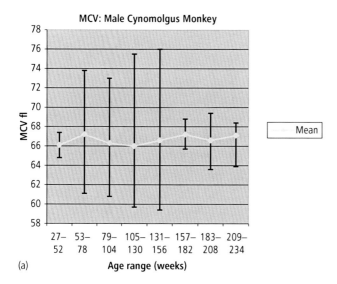

(a)

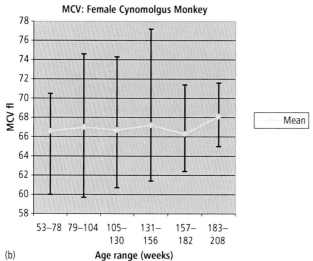

(b)

Figure 5.3 Cynomolgus: mean cell volume (MCV). Male (a) and female (b) animals.

Figure 5.4 Cynomolgus: mean cell hemoglobin concentration (MCHC). Male (a) and female (b) animals.

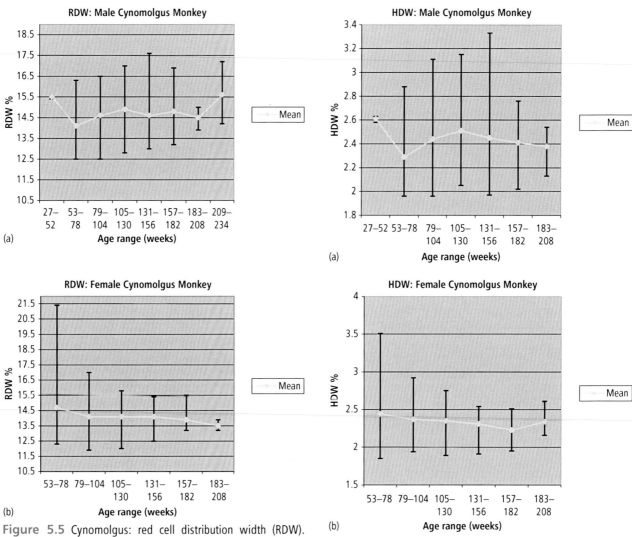

(a)

(b)

Figure 5.5 Cynomolgus: red cell distribution width (RDW). Male (a) and female (b) animals.

Figure 5.6 Cynomolgus: hemoglobin distribution width (HDW). Male (a) and female (b) animals.

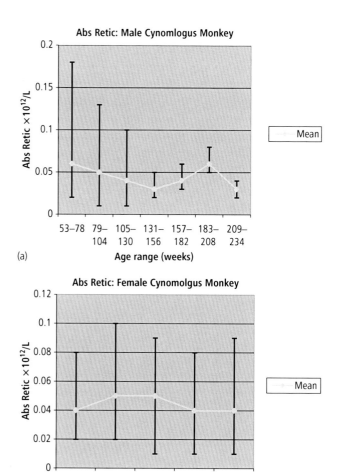

(a)

(b)

Figure 5.7 Cynomolgus: absolute reticulocyte count (Retic Abs). Male (a) and female (b) animals.

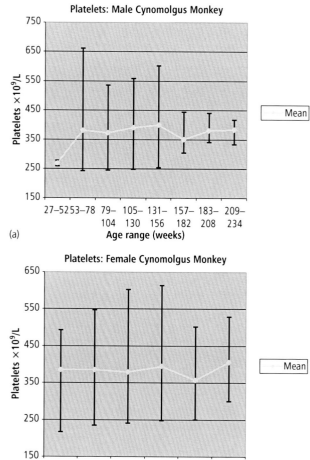

(a)

(b)

Figure 5.8 Cynomolgus: platelet count (PLT). Male (a) and female (b) animals.

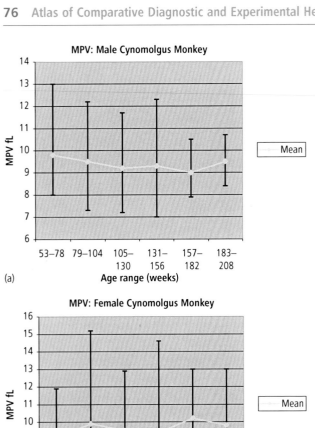

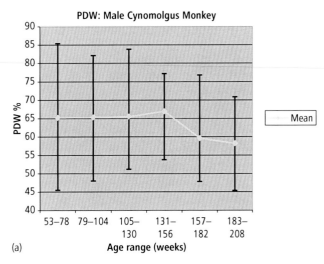

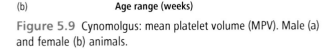

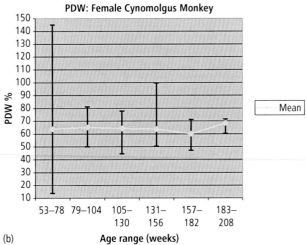

Figure 5.9 Cynomolgus: mean platelet volume (MPV). Male (a) and female (b) animals.

Figure 5.10 Cynomolgus: platelet distribution width (PDW). Male (a) and female (b) animals.

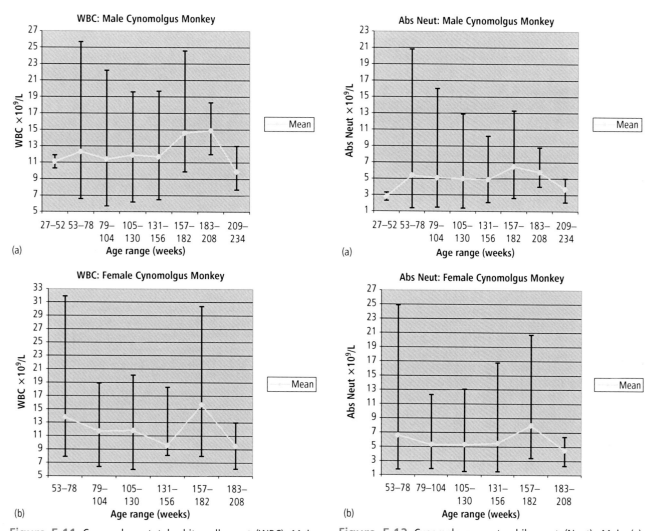

Figure 5.11 Cynomolgus: total white cell count (WBC). Male (a) and female (b) animals.

Figure 5.12 Cynomolgus: neutrophil count (Neut). Male (a) and female (b) animals.

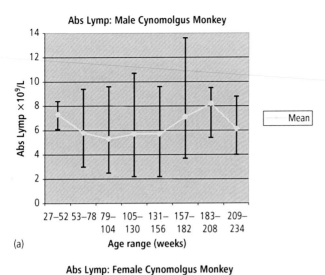

(a)

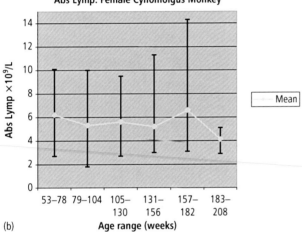

(b)

Figure 5.13 Cynomolgus: lymphocyte count (Lymph). Male (a) and female (b) animals.

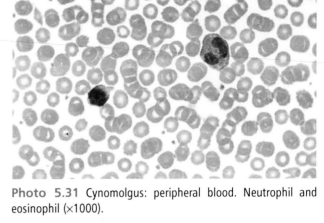

Photo 5.31 Cynomolgus: peripheral blood. Neutrophil and eosinophil (×1000).

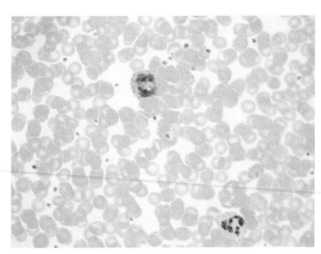

Photo 5.32 Cynomolgus: peripheral blood. Neutrophil and basophil (×1000).

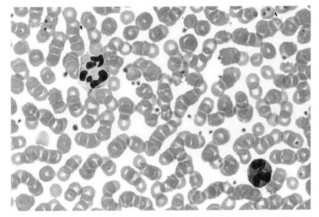

Photo 5.30 Cynomolgus: peripheral blood. Neutrophil and eosinophil. Though there are variations in staining intensity and colour, eosinophils are readily identified microscopically (×1000).

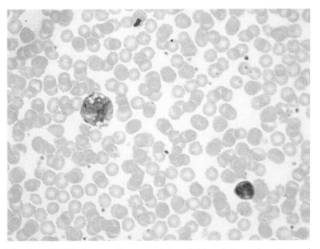

Photo 5.33 Cynomolgus: peripheral blood. Lymphocyte and vacuolated monocyte (×1000).

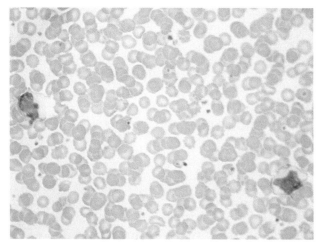

Photo 5.34 Cynomolgus: peripheral blood. Atypical lymphocytes (×1000).

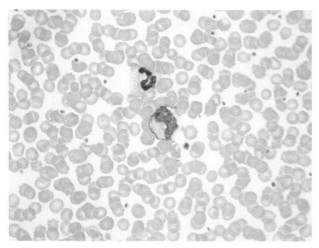

Photo 5.35 Cynomolgus: peripheral blood. Neutrophil and atypical monocyte (×1000).

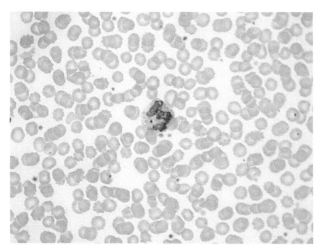

Photo 5.36 Cynomolgus: peripheral blood. Degranulated basophil (×1000).

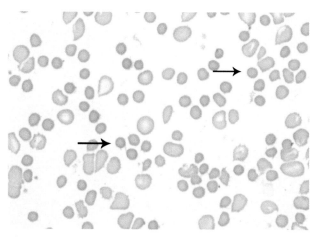

Photo 5.37 Cynomolgus: peripheral blood. Hemolytic anemia: spherocytes (arrowed) (×500).

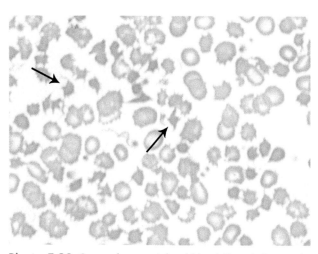

Photo 5.38 Cynomolgus: peripheral blood. Hemolytic anemia: schistocytes (arrowed) (×500).

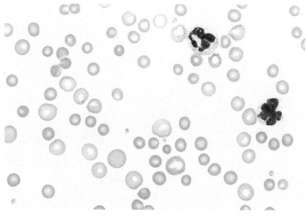

Photo 5.39 Cynomolgus: peripheral blood. Anisocytosis and polychromasia (×1000).

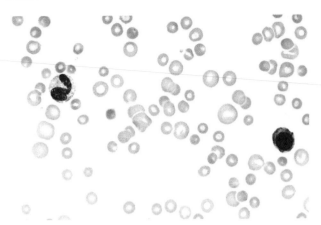

Photo 5.40 Cynomolgus: peripheral blood. Anisocytosis and polychromasia (×1000).

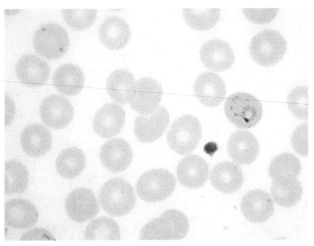

Photo 5.43 Cynomolgus: peripheral blood. *Plasmodium falciparum* (×1000).

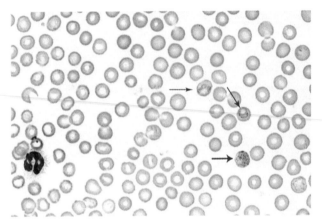

Photo 5.41 Cynomolgus: peripheral blood. *Plasmodium cynomolgi* (arrowed) (×1000).

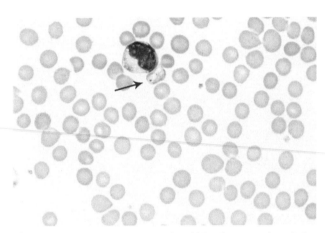

Photo 5.44 Cynomolgus: peripheral blood. Herpesvirus simiae B virus (arrowed) (×1000).

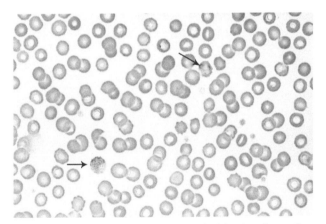

Photo 5.42 Cynomolgus: peripheral blood. *Plasmodium cynomolgi* (arrowed) (×1000).

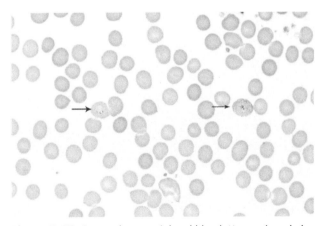

Photo 5.45 Cynomolgus: peripheral blood. Herpesvirus simiae B virus (arrowed) (×1000).

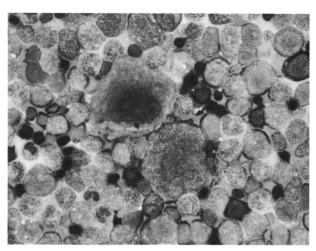

Photo 5.46 Cynomolgus: bone marrow. Healthy animal (×1000).

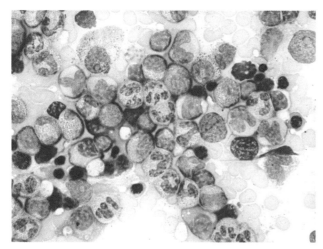

Photo 5.47 Cynomolgus: bone marrow. Healthy animal (×1000).

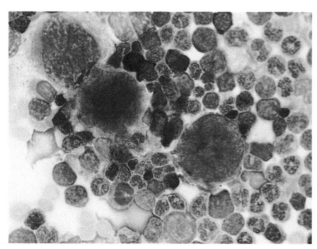

Photo 5.48 Cynomolgus: bone marrow. Reticulum cell and megakaryocyte (×1000).

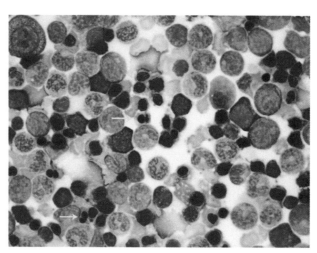

Photo 5.49 Cynomolgus: bone marrow. Reticulum cell and megakaryocyte (×1000).

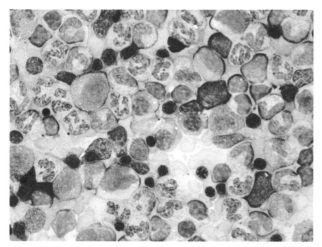

Photo 5.50 Cynomolgus: bone marrow. Dyserythropoesis: binucleated erythroblasts (arrowed) (×1000).

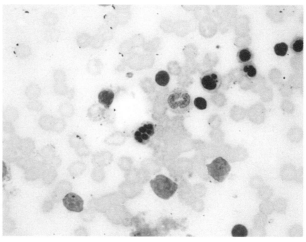

Photo 5.51 Cynomolgus: bone marrow. Dyserythropoesis: multi-nucleated erythroblasts (×1000).

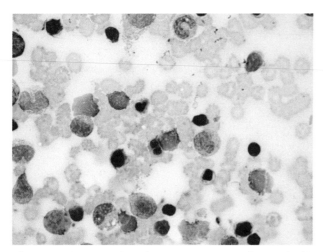

Photo 5.52 Cynomolgus: bone marrow. Dyserythropoesis: bi-nucleated erythroblasts (×1000).

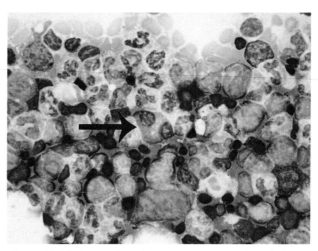

Photo 5.55 Cynomolgus: bone marrow. Bi-nucleated plasma cell (arrowed) (×1000).

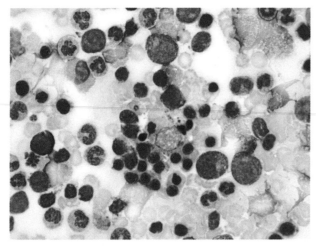

Photo 5.53 Cynomolgus: bone marrow. Healthy animal; erythroblast island (×1000).

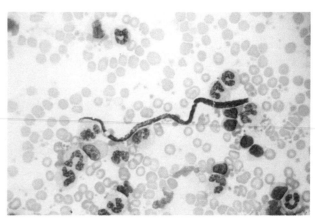

Photo 5.56 Cynomolgus: peripheral blood. *Dirofilaria immitis* (×500).

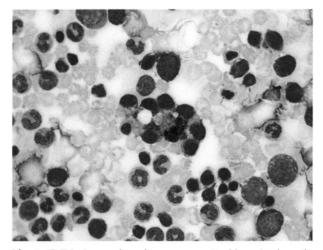

Photo 5.54 Cynomolgus: bone marrow. Healthy animal; erythroblast island (×1000).

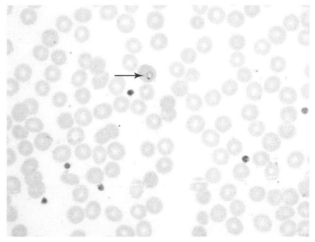

Photo 5.57 Cynomolgus: peripheral blood. Malaria with classic ring form (arrowed) (×500).

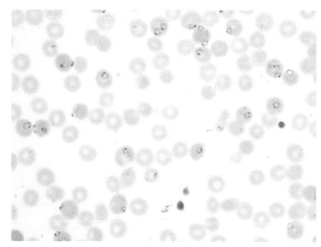

Photo 5.58 Cynomolgus: peripheral blood. Malaria (×500).

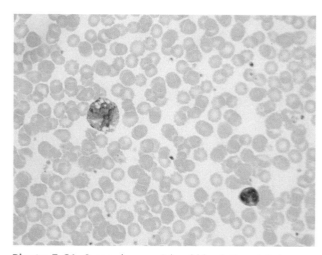

Photo 5.61 Cynomolgus: peripheral blood. Vacuolated mono-cyte (×500).

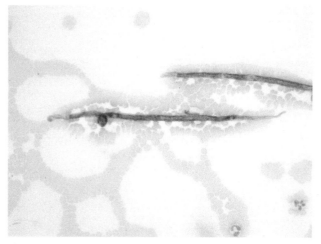

Photo 5.59 Cynomolgus: peripheral blood. Microfilaria (×500).

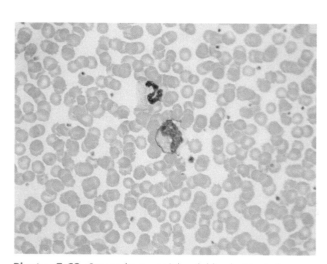

Photo 5.62 Cynomolgus: peripheral blood. Atypical mono-cytes (×500).

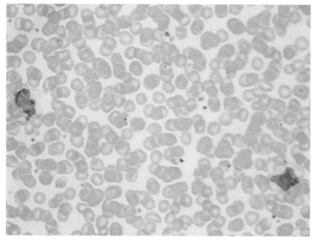

Photo 5.60 Cynomolgus: peripheral blood. Atypical lym-phocytes (×500).

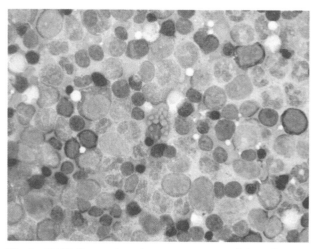

Photo 5.63 Cynomolgus: bone marrow. Fat cell (×500).

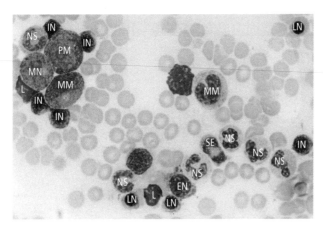

Photo 5.64 Cynomolgus: normal bone marrow. Key: IN, intermediate normoblast; LN, late normoblast; PM, promyelocyte; MN, myelocyte neutrophil; MM, neutrophil metamyelocyte; SE, segmented eosinophil; NS, non-segmented neutrophil; SN, segmented neutrophil; B, basophil; MC, monocyte; L, lymphocyte (×1000).

BABOON

Baboons are rarely encountered in toxicology now but may be encountered in veterinary medicine. A few photos are presented here for comparative purposes.

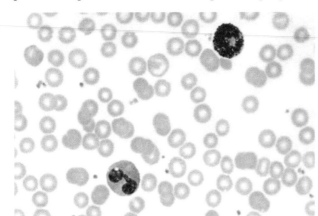

Photo 5.66 Healthy baboon: peripheral blood. Neutrophil and basophil (×1000).

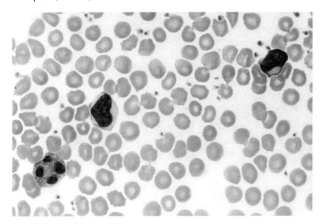

Photo 5.68 Healthy baboon: peripheral blood. Neutrophil and lymphocytes (×1000).

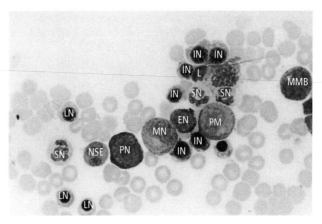

Photo 5.65 Cynomolgus: normal bone marrow. Key: IN, intermediate normoblast; LN, late normoblast; MN, myelocyte neutrophil; PM, promyelocyte; MMB, basophil metamyelocyte; NSE, non-segmented eosinophil; NS, non-segmented neutrophil; L, lymphocyte (×1000).

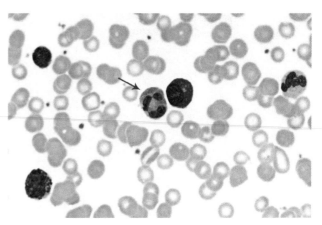

Photo 5.67 Healthy baboon: peripheral blood. Normal neutrophil, basophil, eosinophil (arrowed) and lymphocyte with a plasma cell (rarely seen in peripheral blood) (×1000).

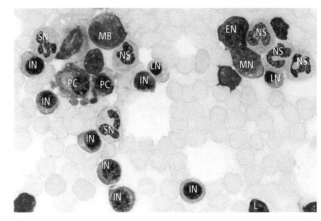

Photo 5.69 Healthy baboon: bone marrow. Key: EN, early normoblast; IN, intermediate normoblast; LN, late normoblast; MB, myeloblast; MN, myelocyte neutrophil; SN, segmented neutrophil; PC, plasma cell; L, lymphocyte; NS, non-segmented neutrophil. (×1000).

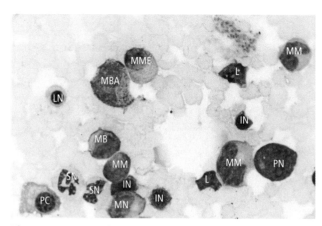

Photo 5.70 Healthy baboon: bone marrow. Key: PN, Pronormoblast; IN, intermediate normoblast; LN, late normoblast; MB, myeloblast; MN, myelocyte neutrophil; MBS, myelocyte basophil; MM, neutrophil metamyelocyte; MME, eosinophil metamyelocyte; SN, segmented neutrophil; PC, plasma cell; L, lymphocyte (×1000).

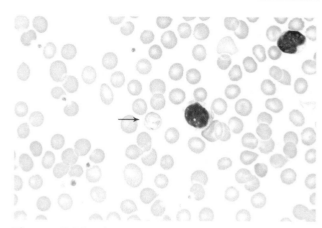

Photo 5.73 Baboon: peripheral blood. Trophozoite of *Hepatocystis simiae* (arrowed) (×1000).

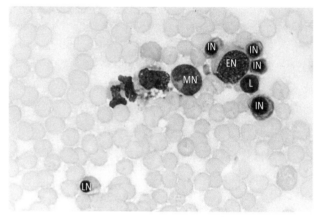

Photo 5.71 Healthy baboon: bone marrow. Key: EN, early normoblast; IN, intermediate normoblast; LN, late normoblast; MN, myelocyte neutrophil; L, lymphocyte (×1000).

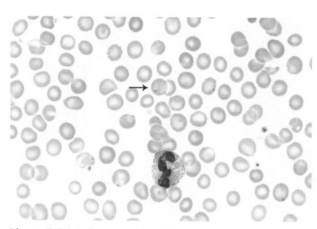

Photo 5.74 Baboon: peripheral blood. Ring form of *Hepatocystis simiae* (arrowed) (×1000).

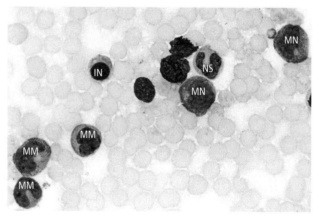

Photo 5.72 Healthy baboon. bone marrow. Key: IN, intermediate normoblast; MM, neutrophil metamyelocyte; MN, myelocyte neutrophil; NS, non-segmented neutrophil (×1000).

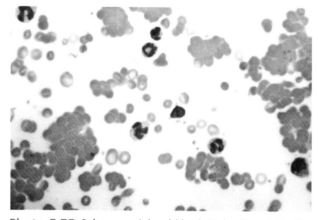

Photo 5.75 Baboon: peripheral blood. Red cell agglutination due to treatment with a novel anti-lymphocyte compound (×1000).

RHESUS MONKEY

Rhesus monkeys are not encountered in toxicology now due to endangerment issues, but may be encountered in veterinary medicine. A few photos are presented here for comparative purposes.

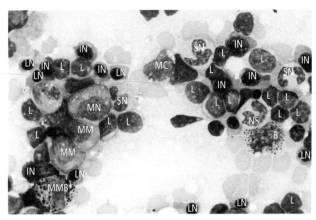

Photo 5.79 Healthy rhesus monkey: bone marrow. Key: IN, intermediate normoblast; LN, late normoblast; MN, myelocyte neutrophil; MM, neutrophil metamyelocyte; MMB, basophil metamyelocyte; NS, non-segmented neutrophil; SN, segmented neutrophil; B, basophil; MC, monocyte; L, lymphocyte (×1000).

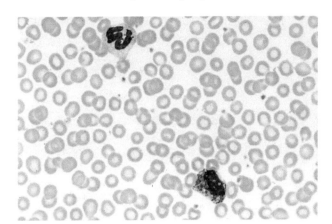

Photo 5.76 Healthy rhesus monkey: peripheral blood. Neutrophil and basophil (×1000).

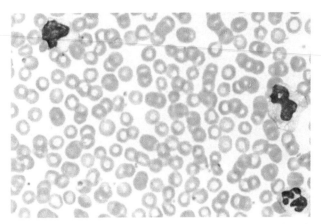

Photo 5.77 Healthy rhesus monkey: peripheral blood. Neutrophil, lymphocyte and vacuolated monocyte (×1000).

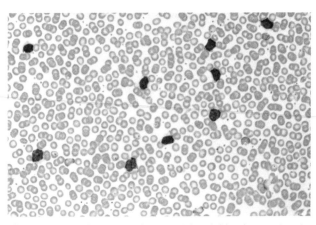

Photo 5.80 Rhesus monkey: peripheral blood. Parasitemia: lymphocytosis (×500).

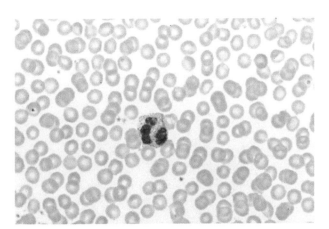

Photo 5.78 Healthy rhesus monkey: peripheral blood. Eosinophil (×1000).

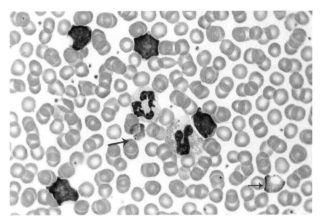

Photo 5.81 Rhesus monkey: peripheral blood. Parasitemia: Neutrophils, lymphocytes and *Hepatocystis* sp. parasites (arrowed) (×500).

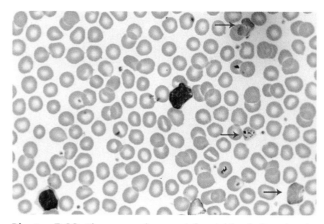

Photo 5.82 Rhesus monkey: peripheral blood. Parasitemia: Lymphocytes and *Hepatocystis* sp. parasites (arrowed) (×1000).

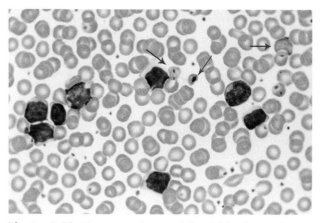

Photo 5.83 Rhesus monkey: peripheral blood. Parasitemia: Lymphocytes and *Hepatocystis* sp. parasites (arrowed) (×1000).

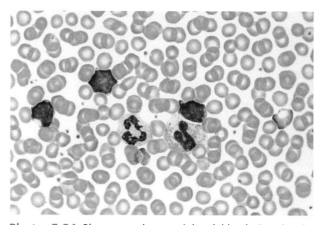

Photo 5.84 Rhesus monkey: peripheral blood. Parasitemia: Neutrophils, lymphocytes and *Hepatocystis* sp. parasites (×1000).

References

1. Scarborough RA (1931–32). The blood picture of normal laboratory animals. A compilation of published data. *Yale J Biol Med* 199 (The monkey).
2. Gardner MV (1947). The blood picture of normal laboratory animals. A review of the literature 1936–1946. *J Franklin Inst* 244: 155 (The Monkey).
3. Feldman BF, Zinkl JG, Jain NC (eds) (2010). *Schalm's Veterinary Hematology (6th edn)*. Baltimore: Lippincott Williams & Wilkins.
4. Shimwell M, Warrington BF, Fowler JSL (1979). Dietary habits relating to "wasting marmoset syndrome" (WMS). *Lab Anim* 13: 139–142.
5. Hawkey CM, Hart MG (1986). Is the presence of Heinz bodies diagnostic for wasting marmoset syndrome? Eighteenth Triennial Conference of the Institute of Medical Laboratory Sciences, Southampton, England. Aug 18–22. *Med Lab Sci* 43 (Suppl.1).
6. Ghebremeskel K, Williams G, Harbige L, *et al.* (1990). Plasma vitamins A and E and hydrogen peroxide-induced in-vitro erythrocyte haemolysis in common marmosets. *Vet Rec* 126: 429–431.
7. Reinhardt V (1997). Training non-human primates to cooperate during blood collection – a review. *Lab Primate Newslett* 36: 1.

6

Other species

Occasionally samples from alternative species are received in the laboratory where domesticated species may be the subject of investigation e.g. for veterinary, ecological or environmental study.

We present here a selection of peripheral blood pictures offered to us for publication as examples of the diversity of animal species sometimes encountered in comparative, diagnostic and experimental work the world over.

Reference data are not provided, but we re-emphasise that typical data ranges should be determined for each laboratory. The use of concurrent (normal) control samples in preclinical work is often used for comparative purposes in determining the health status of individuals or groups of animals: where veterinary examination is required it is useful to obtain samples from a companion animal.

PIG

Introduction

Most hematological parameters in the pig are influenced by the age of the animal and normal values vary greatly between strains. This is less so for specific pathogen free (SPF) -derived or minimal disease (MD) pigs, which are increasingly used in toxicology as a non-rodent alternative to the dog. These pigs have been bred as miniature animals and several strains are widely available.

Blood picture

Generally, red cell parameters are similar to those of humans although vary with breed, growth rate, age, diet, stage of gestation/lactation, feeding method, management practices and season[1]. Red cells readily form rouleaux and rapidly undergo spontaneous crenation shortly after collection, presumably (as in rodents), due to decreased levels of intracellular ATP. Anisocytosis is common along with large polychromatic cells, nucleated red cells and occasional Howell–Jolly Bodies.

Total white cell counts of SPF and MD strains are lower than those of conventional pigs, the lymphocyte being the predominant leukocyte. Neutrophil, eosinophil and basophil numbers tend to be relatively high in conventional pigs when compared to SPF varieties, and an increase in neutrophils is widely regarded as being a reliable indicator of SPF status breakdown.

Morphologically, cells of SPF-derived strains do not differ appreciably from those of conventional varieties, although monocytes can be difficult to identify correctly, possibly accounting for the wide ranges reported in the literature. Band neutrophils may be present in healthy animals, earlier forms having a ring nucleus; eosinophils may also appear immature. Basophils have dumbbell-shaped granules.

Platelet volumes are more consistent than those of rat, dog and monkey, although numbers can be quite variable due to spontaneous clumping.

Atlas of Comparative Diagnostic and Experimental Hematology, Second Edition. Clifford Smith, Alfred Jarecki.
© 2011 Blackwell Publishing Ltd. Published 2011 by Blackwell Publishing Ltd.

Table 6.1 Blood parameters of mini-pigs (Siemens Advia 120).

Minipig	Units	Male			Female		
		Min	Mean	Max	Min	Mean	Max
Hb	g/dL	11.9	13.7	15.6	12.0	13.4	14.8
RBC	x10⁶/µL	8.45	6.87	9.72	7.96	6.80	8.99
MCV	fL	40.8	48.1	58.1	41.8	48.0	58.9
MCHC	g/dL	32.0	33.9	35.7	29.8	33.5	35.5
Retics	x10⁶/µL	60	195	410	90	238	375
Plts	x10³/µL	356	622	917	280	628	1052
WBC	x10³/µL	5.9	11.4	24.3	6.1	11.8	18.4
Neuts	x10³/µL	1.4	4.8	15.5	0.6	3.2	8.3
Lymphs	x10³/µL	4.0	5.8	8.6	4.5	7.5	12.2

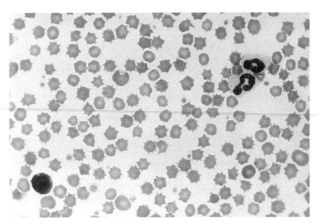

Photo 6.1 Healthy mini-pig: peripheral blood. Crenation, two neutrophils and a lymphocyte (×1000).

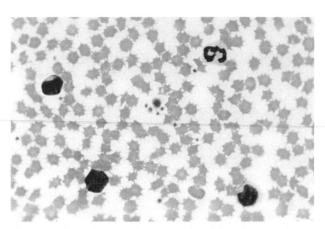

Photo 6.2 Healthy mini-pig: peripheral blood. Crenation, a neutrophil, two lymphocytes and a basophil (×1000).

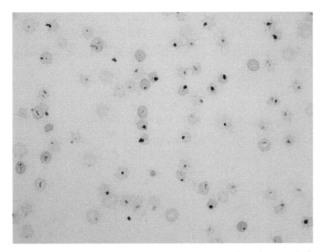

Photo 6.3 Mini-pig: peripheral blood. Treated with a methyl-thioninium compound. Methyl violet stain (84% Heinz bodies) (×1000).

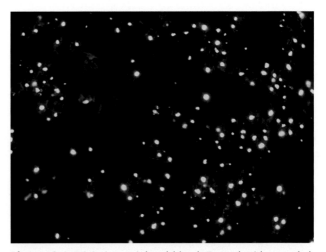

Photo 6.4 Mini-pig: peripheral blood. Treated with a methyl-thioninium compound, demonstrating Heinz Bodies stained *in-vivo*. PB. Phenyl Auramine: fluorescent microscopy (×100).

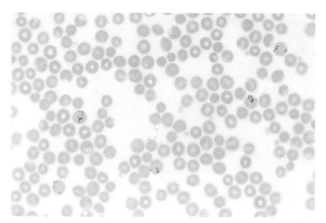

Photo 6.5 Mini-pig: peripheral blood. Treated with a methylthioninium compound demonstrating *in vivo* reticulocyte staining (×1000).

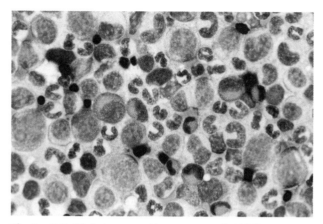

Photo 6.7 Mini-pig: normal bone marrow (×1000).

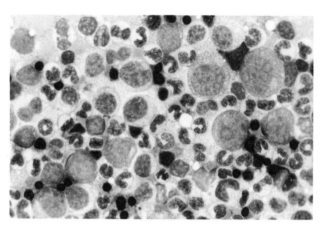

Photo 6.6 Mini-pig: normal bone marrow (×1000).

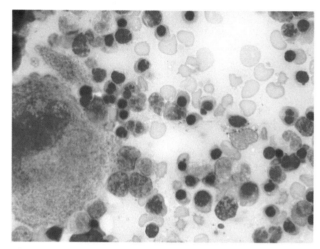

Photo 6.8 Mini-pig: bone marrow. Erythroid hyperplasia (×1000).

HORSE

Introduction

The horse (*Equus caballus*) and donkey/burro (*Equus asinus*) can be employed as large-scale reservoirs for the production of antisera; they are seldom encountered in toxicology unless safety evaluation is being performed on a drug intended for equine use. The blood presents some interesting and distinctive features which are worth noting.

Blood picture

Thoroughbreds derived from Arab stock ("hot-blooded" horses) generally have appreciably higher erythrocyte parameters than draughthorses, ponies and similar varieties ("cold-blooded" varieties), and the mean corpuscular volume (MCV) is often smaller[2]. There are few other hematological differences, although reticulocytes are conspicuously absent from the circulation. Erythrocytes form rouleaux very readily producing an elevated erythrocyte sedimentation rate (ESR), as high as 90 mm in the first hour. Exercise and excitement generally increase the circulating red cell mass and leukocyte count by up to 20% from splenic contraction. Total white cell counts are more variable in the hot-blooded horse than the cold-blooded variety.

Neutrophil, lymphocyte, monocyte and basophil morphology is unremarkable. The eosinophil is distinctive, filled with granules to the point where the cytoplasmic membrane literally bulges and the nucleus is obscured.

Platelet counts (similar to those of humans), volume estimations (very much smaller than human platelets) and population statistics may be compromised by clumping of platelets even in EDTA. Platelet count validity must be considered very carefully in the light of microscopic examination of the blood smear.

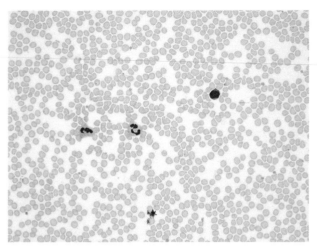

Photo 6.9 Horse: peripheral blood. Neutrophils and lymphocyte (×500).

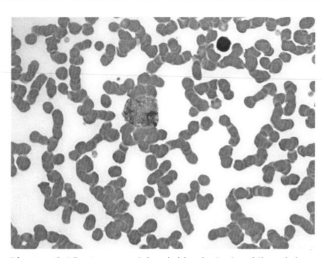

Photo 6.12 Horse: peripheral blood. Eosinophil and lymphocyte (×1000).

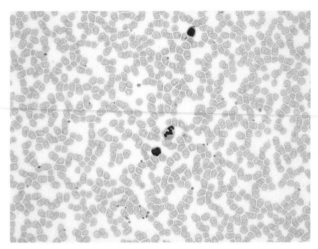

Photo 6.10 Horse: peripheral blood. Neutrophil and lymphocytes. Red cells demonstrate rouleaux (×500).

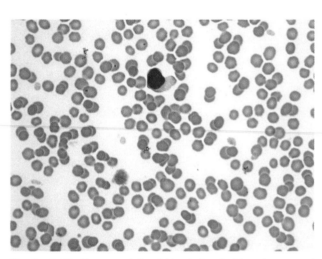

Photo 6.13 Horse: peripheral blood. Atypical lymphocyte and large platelet (×1000).

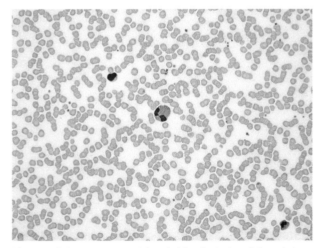

Photo 6.11 Horse: peripheral blood. Eosinophil and lymphocyte. Red cells demonstrate rouleaux (×500).

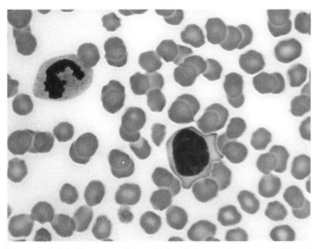

Photo 6.14 Horse: peripheral blood. Agranular neutrophil and reactive lymphocyte (×1000).

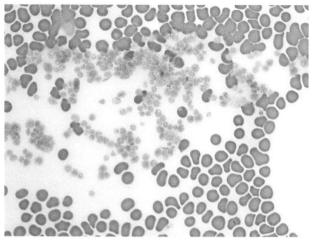

Photo 6.15 Horse: peripheral blood. Aggregated platelets (×1000).

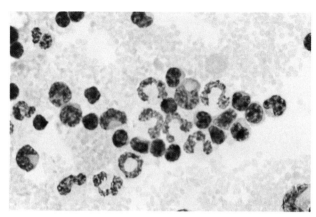

Photo 6.18 Horse: bone marrow. Normal (×1000).

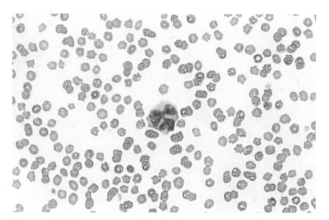

Photo 6.16 Horse: peripheral blood. Clover-leaf lymphosarcoma (×1000).

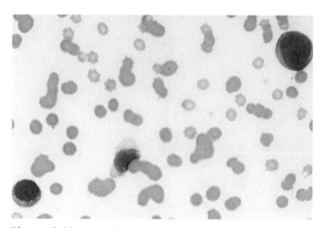

Photo 6.19 Horse: bone marrow. Lymphoma (×1000).

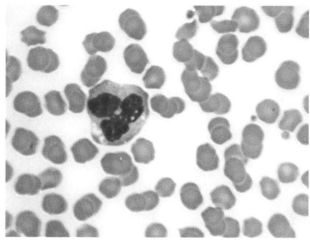

Photo 6.17 Horse: peripheral blood. Clover-leaf lymphosarcoma (×1000).

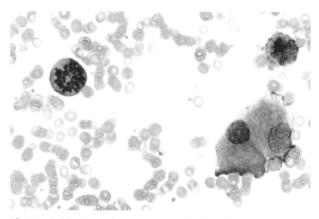

Photo 6.20 Horse: bone marrow. Mitotic cell and plasma cells (×1000).

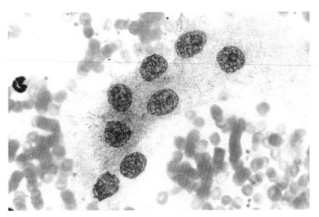

Photo 6.21 Horse: bone marrow. Osteoclasts (×1000).

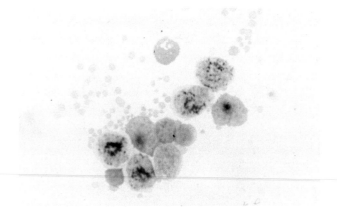

Photo 6.22 Horse: bone marrow. Myelo-monocytic differentiation demonstrated by this dual esterase stain (×1000).

GOAT AND SHEEP

Goats and sheep are occasionally encountered in metabolic, environmental and veterinary work. A small selection of photographs is presented here for comparative purposes.

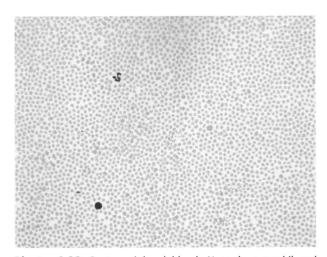

Photo 6.23 Goat: peripheral blood. Normal neutrophil and lymphocyte. Note the aggregation of platelets (×500).

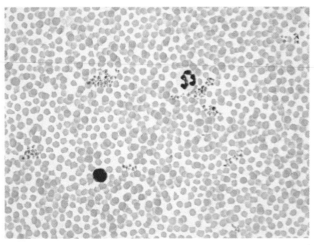

Photo 6.24 Goat: peripheral blood. Normal neutrophil and lymphocyte. Note the aggregation of platelets (×1000).

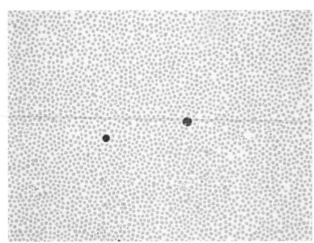

Photo 6.25 Goat: peripheral blood. Normal lymphocytes. (×500).

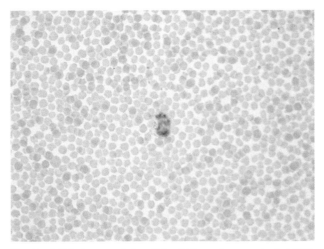

Photo 6.26 Goat: peripheral blood. Normal monocyte. (×1000).

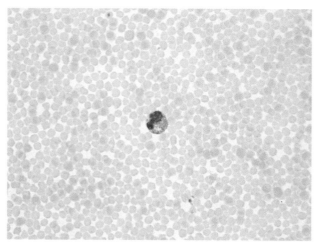

Photo 6.27 Goat: peripheral blood. Normal eosinophil (×1000).

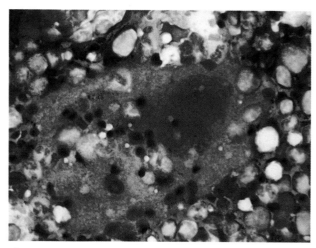

Photo 6.30 Goat: normal bone marrow. (×1000).

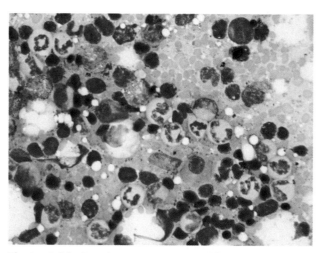

Photo 6.28 Goat: bone marrow. Normal (×1000).

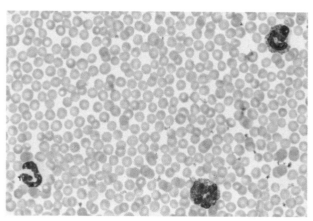

Photo 6.31 Sheep: peripheral blood. Normal neutrophil and two eosinophils (×1000).

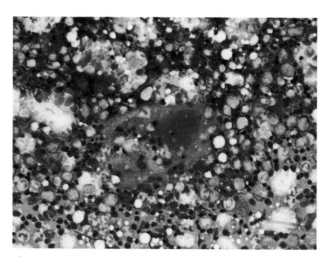

Photo 6.29 Goat: bone marrow. Normal (×500).

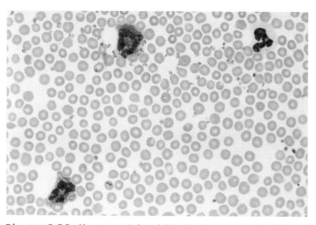

Photo 6.32 Sheep: peripheral blood. Normal neutrophil and two eosinophils (×1000).

ASSORTED OTHER SPECIES

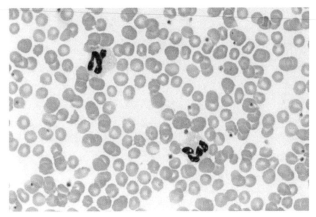

Photo 6.33 Healthy ferret: peripheral blood. Neutrophils (×1000).

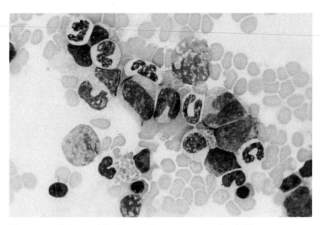

Photo 6.36 Healthy ferret: bone marrow (×1000).

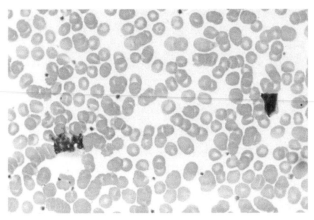

Photo 6.34 Healthy ferret: peripheral blood. Lymphocyte and monocyte (×1000).

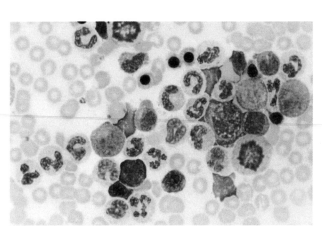

Photo 6.37 Healthy ferret: bone marrow (×1000).

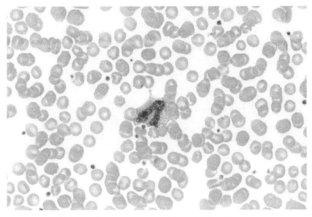

Photo 6.35 Healthy ferret: peripheral blood. Immature neutrophil (×1000).

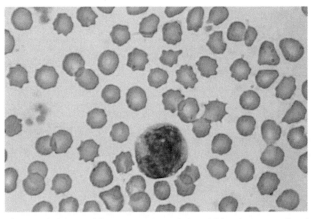

Photo 6.38 Healthy opossum: peripheral blood. Crenated red cells and myelocyte (×1000).

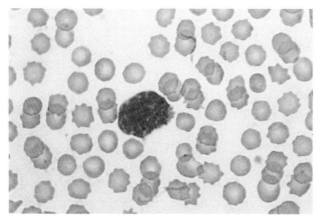

Photo 6.39 Healthy opossum: peripheral blood. Crenated red cells and toxic myelocyte (×1000).

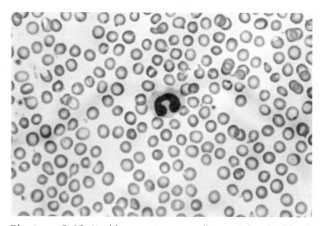

Photo 6.42 Healthy eastern quoll: peripheral blood. Anisocytosis and band cell (×1000).

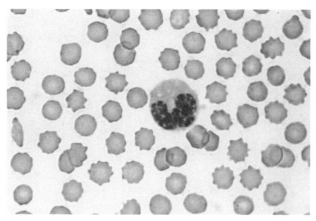

Photo 6.40 Healthy opossum: peripheral blood. Crenated red cells and band cell (×1000).

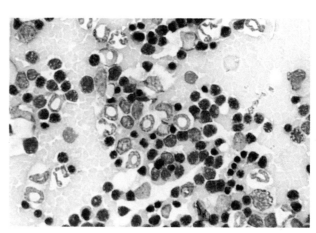

Photo 6.43 Healthy eastern quoll: bone marrow. (×1000).

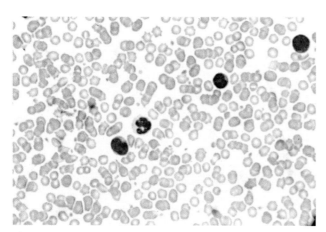

Photo 6.41 Healthy eastern quoll: peripheral blood. Neutrophil and lymphocytes (×500).

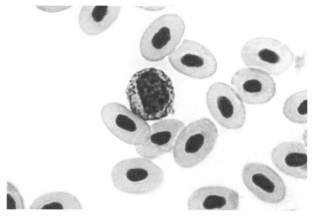

Photo 6.44 Little penguin: peripheral blood. Nucleated erythrocytes and a heterophil (×1000).

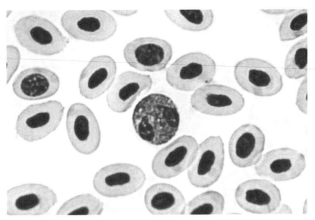

Photo 6.45 Little penguin: peripheral blood. Nucleated erythrocytes and a heterophil (×1000).

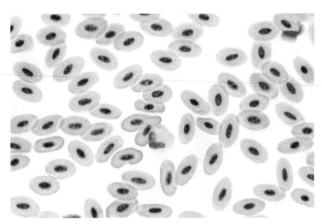

Photo 6.48 Little penguin: peripheral blood. Nucleated erythrocytes and heterophil (×1000).

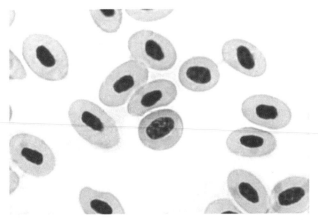

Photo 6.46 Little penguin: peripheral blood. Nucleated erythrocytes and a juvenile red cell (×1000).

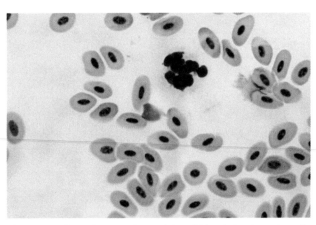

Photo 6.49 Little penguin: peripheral blood. Nucleated erythrocytes and broken heterophil nucleus (×1000).

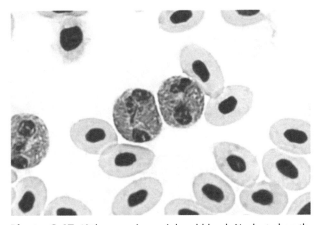

Photo 6.47 Little penguin: peripheral blood. Nucleated erythrocytes and heterophils (×1000).

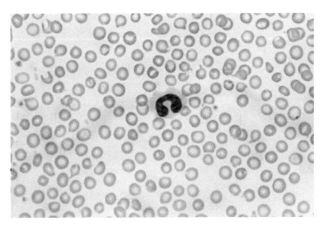

Photo 6.50 Southern elephant seal: peripheral blood (×1000).

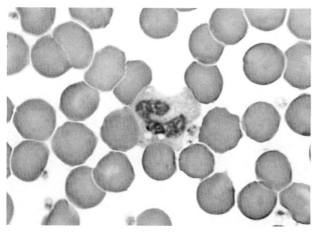

Photo 6.51 Southern elephant seal: peripheral blood (×1000).

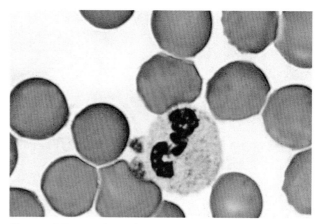

Photo 6.54 Southern elephant seal: peripheral blood, neutrophil (×1000).

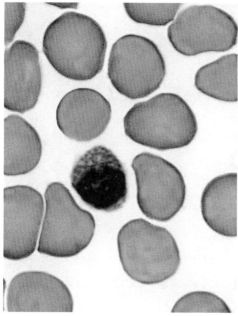

Photo 6.52 Southern elephant seal: peripheral blood, lymphocyte (×1000).

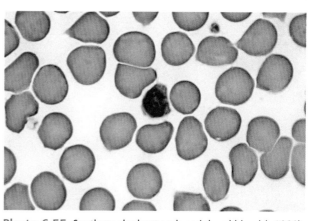

Photo 6.55 Southern elephant seal: peripheral blood (×1000).

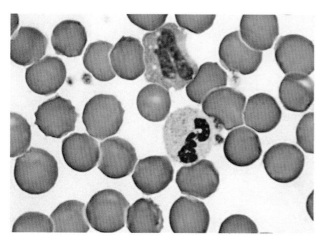

Photo 6.53 Southern elephant seal: peripheral blood (×1000).

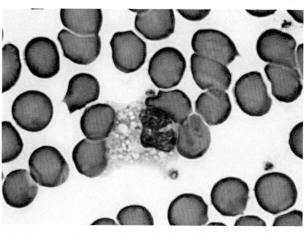

Photo 6.56 Southern elephant seal: peripheral blood (×1000).

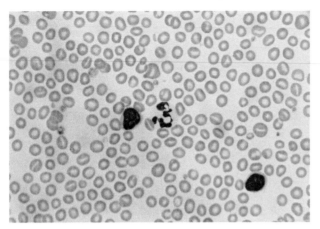

Photo 6.57 Southern hairy-nosed wombat: peripheral blood (×1000).

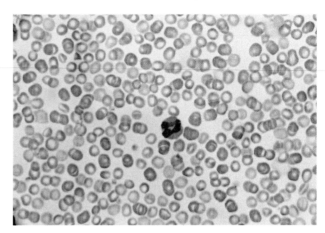

Photo 6.60 Southern hairy-nosed wombat: peripheral blood (×1000).

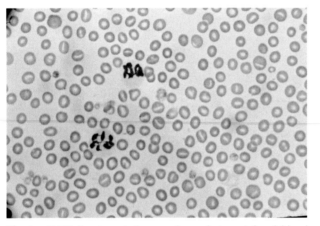

Photo 6.58 Southern hairy-nosed wombat: peripheral blood (×1000).

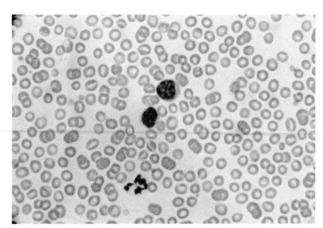

Photo 6.61 Southern hairy-nosed wombat: peripheral blood (×1000).

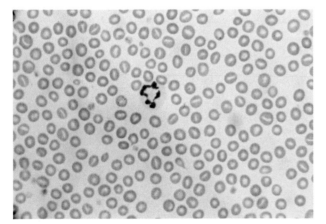

Photo 6.59 Southern hairy-nosed wombat: peripheral blood (×1000).

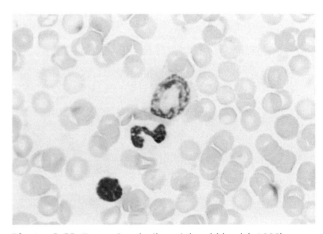

Photo 6.62 Tasmanian devil: peripheral blood (×1000).

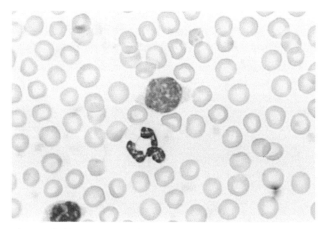

Photo 6.63 Tasmanian devil: peripheral blood (×1000).

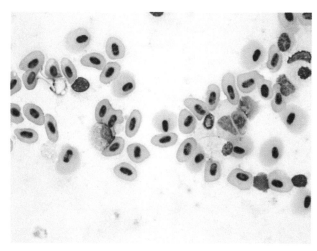

Photo 6.66 Carp: peripheral blood (×1000).

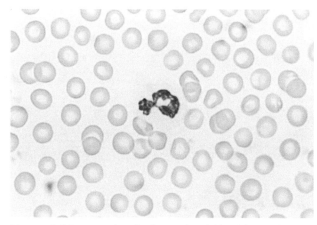

Photo 6.64 Tasmanian devil: peripheral blood (×1000).

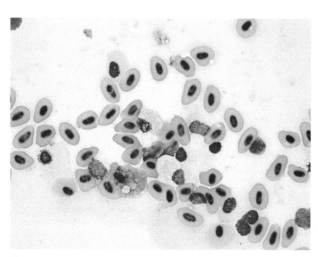

Photo 6.67 Carp: peripheral blood (×1000).

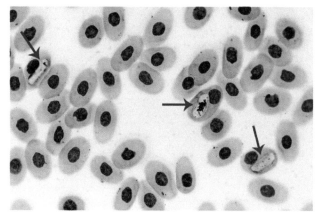

Photo 6.65 Tortoise: peripheral blood. *Haemogangarina* (arrowed) (×1000).

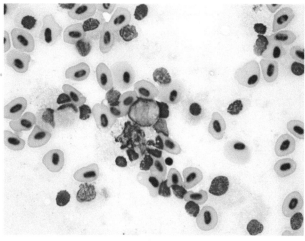

Photo 6.68 Carp: peripheral blood (×1000).

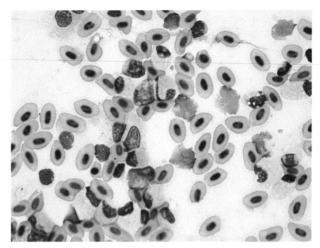

Photo 6.69 Carp: peripheral blood (×1000).

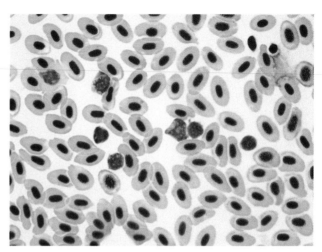

Photo 6.72 Rainbow trout: peripheral blood (×1000).

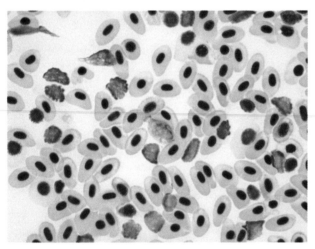

Photo 6.70 Carp: peripheral blood (×1000).

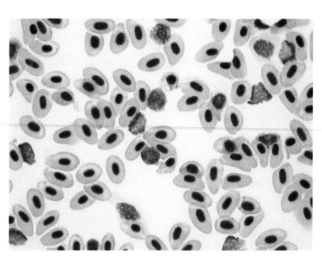

Photo 6.73 Rainbow trout: peripheral blood (×1000).

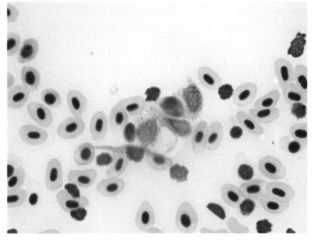

Photo 6.71 Rainbow trout: peripheral blood (×1000).

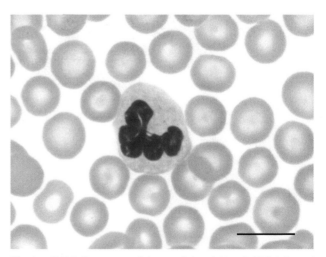

Photo 6.74 Tammar wallaby: peripheral blood. Wright's and Giemsa stain. Normal red cells and neutrophil. Scale bar = 10 μm.

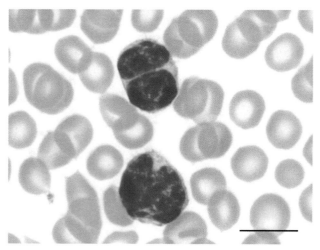

Photo 6.75 Tammar wallaby: peripheral blood. Wright's and Giemsa stain. Normal red cells and lymphocytes which have cleaved nuclei, almost appearing binucleate, a very thin strand of DNA connecting the two hemispheres. Scale bar = 10 μm.

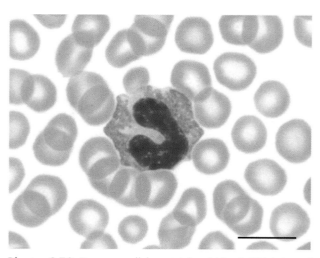

Photo 6.78 Tammar wallaby: peripheral blood. Wright's and Giemsa stain. Normal red cells and eosinophil. Scale bar = 10 μm.

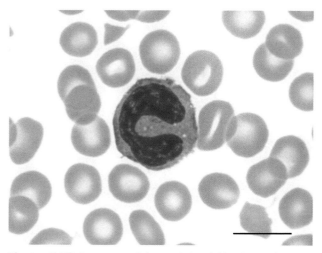

Photo 6.76 Tammar wallaby: peripheral blood. Wright's and Giemsa stain. Normal red cells and monocyte. Scale bar = 10 μm.

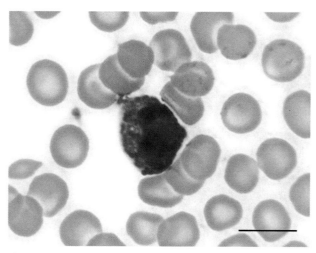

Photo 6.79 Tammar wallaby: peripheral blood. Wright's and Giemsa stain. A basophil – rare in this species. Scale bar = 10 μm.

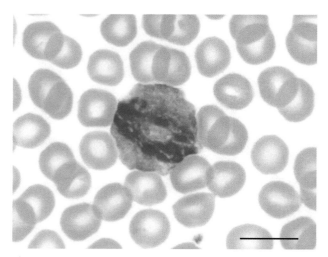

Photo 6.77 Tammar wallaby: peripheral blood. Wright's and Giemsa stain. Normal red cells and an eosinophil, granulocytes occasionally having ring-form nuclei. Scale bar = 10 μm.

References

1. Feldman BF, Zinkl JG, Jain NC (eds) (2010). *Schalm's Veterinary Hematology (6th edn)*. Baltimore: Lippincott Williams & Wilkins.
2. Satue K, Blanco O, Munoz A (2009). Age-related differences in the haematological profile of Andalusian broodmares of Carthusian strain. *Vet Med (Praha)* 4: 175–182.

7

Blood collection procedures

For most large species blood is collected using a needle and syringe or vacuum technique governed by the size of animal and the volume of blood required. Where repeated samples are required there are advantages associated with taking blood from one site only; for example, proficiency with one regularly used technique will improve sample quality. Consistency in bleeding technique and site means that data will be comparable with those obtained at different time points; different bleeding sites may produce differing cell counts masking dynamic changes in cell numbers. It is therefore critical for a laboratory to establish its own typical ranges using its preferred bleeding site, method of collection, analytical methods, etc.

Common bleeding sites

Rodents present special problems because of their small blood vessels. Retro-orbital sinus bleeds have been a popular site of choice, while tail vein bleeds on restrained unanesthetised animals are now more common. Cleaning of the tail is important to avoid contamination of the sample by epidermal cells or bacteria. Tail transection will provide little more blood than is sufficient for a blood film. Cardiac puncture has been used where larger volumes are required, although this method should be reserved for post-mortem collection.

The preferred venipuncture site for rabbits is an ear vein. Dogs are conveniently phlebotomised from the jugular vein, although the cephalic vein is also used. Primates are conveniently phlebotomised from the femoral vein.

Table 7.1 lists commonly used sites. Hazards include the use of anesthesia, accidental collection of mixtures of arterial and venous blood and tissue fluid contamination. The quality of the samples is especially dependent on the care taken during collection.

Anticoagulants

Once blood has been obtained it must be transferred immediately to an anticoagulant if cell counts or morphology are to be examined. For routine hematology cell counts and blood films, di-potassium or tri-potassium salts of EDTA are preferred; other anticoagulants should be avoided for routine cell morphology due to artifactual changes, e.g. platelet clumping, dilution, background staining, etc. Heparinised syringes may be of help and induce minimal morphological changes in obtaining samples from slow-bleeding animals.

Staining

Romanowsky stains, used for most of the illustrations in this atlas, are appropriate for most species without modification. Leishman's, modified Wright's, Jenner's and May–Grünwald–Giemsa stains are equally suitable; personal preference will dictate which particular stain is used for routine examinations. Correct fixation and staining are important and critical to the interpretation of abnormalities. Where abnormalities are flagged by an automatic analyser it will be necessary to examine a manually prepared blood film stained by conventional techniques for confirmation.

Atlas of Comparative Diagnostic and Experimental Hematology, Second Edition. Clifford Smith, Alfred Jarecki.
© 2011 Blackwell Publishing Ltd. Published 2011 by Blackwell Publishing Ltd.

Table 7.1 Common blood collection sites.

Blood collection site	Species									
	Mouse	Hamster	Guinea pig	Rat	Rabbit	Dog	Cat	Mini-pig	Monkey	Horse/cow
Tail vein	–	–	–	#	–	–	–	–	–	–
Tail transection*	#	–	–	#	–	–	–	–	–	–
Sublingual	–	–	–	#	–	–	–	–	–	–
Abdominal aorta**	#	#	#	#	–	–	–	–	–	–
Retro-orbital sinus	–	–	–	#	–	–	–	–	–	–
Cardiac puncture**	#	#	#	#	–	–	–	–	–	–
Jugular vein	–	–	–	#	#	#	–	#	#	#
Cephalic vein	–	–	–	–	–	#	#	–	–	–
Marginal ear vein	–	–	–	–	#	–	–	–	–	–
Femoral vein	–	–	–	–	–	–	–	–	#	–

*Useful for blood smear preparation only.
**At termination.

8

Artifacts

An artifact is defined as "something in a biological specimen that is not present naturally but has been introduced or produced during a procedure"[1]. Artifacts can be induced pre-collection and during collection, storage and/or preparation, causing specific and/or non-specific changes to cell morphology.

Even before a sample is collected artifacts may include numerical, morphological or functional changes, e.g. dehydration will elevate cell counts due to hemoconcentration; undue stress during animal handling may cause an artificial rise in total white cell count due to granulocyte demargination. Marginating cells are rapidly swept from blood vessel endothelia into the lumen by endogenous or exogenous epinephrine as a result of exercise or as a result of a rapid increase in cardiac output. These responses can double neutrophil counts very quickly, and are reversible equally quickly. Good husbandry and experienced, confident operators are therefore crucial to the quality and integrity of the sample being collected.

Hematology data must be interpreted in the light of typical ranges generated in the same laboratory, as this is dependent on many variables, e.g. strain, age, sex, collection site, methodology, and many other physical and biological factors[2]. This is particularly important for rodent species due to the special considerations for blood collection, such as age and size of the animal, and the ability to collect a suitable quantity and quality of sample. Within 24 hours of sample collection horse platelets clump and appear in the eosinophil area of the cytogram on automated flow cytometers, leading to inaccurate platelet counts and white cell differentials.

Sex differences are demonstrable in erythrocyte, leukocyte and platelet counts, which are generally higher in male than female animals in most species.

Exercise and stress may increase erythrocyte and leukocyte counts through the requirements for increased oxygen carrying capacity[3] and as a defence mechanism. It is necessary therefore to reduce stress to an animal during blood collection, and to ensure that a "clean" and consistent technique is used. This is especially important in toxicological evaluation where treated subjects may be compared to concurrent controls, previous data generated for that study (individual data and group means) and possibly in combination with, or in addition to, background or reference data.

Fasting for 17–20 hours causes a moderate increase in erythrocyte count, hemoglobin and hematocrit, and a distinct decrease in leukocyte count[4].

Collection artifacts

Different blood collection sites may affect values obtained. In our laboratory, for example, rat erythrocyte counts and hemoglobin are highest in jugular blood, whereas total white cell and lymphocyte counts are highest from orbital sinus samples.

However, total leukocyte counts, hemoglobin and hematocrit are reported in the literature to be highest in peripheral samples taken by tail vein bleed and lowest from arterial samples[5].

A common difficulty in toxicological studies occurs where many samples are being collected, for example studies in rodents usually involve more than two to

Table 8.1 Red cell variation related to blood collection site.

	Male rat			Female rat	
Collection site	Mean RBC ($\times 10^{12}$/L)	Mean HB (g/dL)	Collection site	Mean RBC ($\times 10^{12}$/L)	Mean HB (g/dL)
Tail vein	7.63	15.1	Tail vein	8.07	15.7
Sublingual	7.54	15.1	Sublingual	7.47	14.6
Jugular	8.63	16.3	Jugular	8.29	15.9
Orbital sinus	7.83	15.3	Orbital sinus	7.74	14.9

Table 8.2 White cell variation related to blood collection site.

	Male rat				Female rat		
Collection site	Mean total white cell count ($\times 10^9$/L)	Mean neutrophil count ($\times 10^9$/L)	Mean lymphocyte count ($\times 10^9$/L)	Collection site	Mean total white cell count ($\times 10^9$/L)	Mean neutrophil count ($\times 10^9$/L)	Mean lymphocyte count ($\times 10^9$/L)
Tail vein	8.60	1.10	7.30	Tail vein	6.20	0.70	5.20
Sublingual	9.80	1.00	8.40	Sublingual	7.10	0.90	6.00
Jugular	8.90	1.20	7.50	Jugular	5.30	0.70	4.40
Orbital sinus	10.50	1.20	8.90	Orbital sinus	7.40	0.80	6.30

Table 8.3 Platelet variation related to blood collection site.

	Male rat				Female rat		
Collection site	Mean PLT ($\times 10^9$/L)	Mean MPV (fL)	Mean PDW (%)	Collection site	Mean PLT ($\times 10^9$/L)	Mean MPV (fL)	Mean PDW (%)
Tail vein	1093	9.8	52.5	Tail vein	1152	9.3	50.6
Sublingual	1058	9.1	51.5	Sublingual	1192	9.0	49.9
Jugular	1107	9.2	52.4	Jugular	1099	8.9	53.6
Orbital sinus	1005	9.0	51.1	Orbital sinus	1039	8.8	53.5

four times as many animals as larger species. The time taken to bleed rodents, especially if procedures are introduced such as prior warming, can mean that it can take a prolonged period of time to collect all samples. In addition, samples collected at post mortem may be spread throughout a full day because of the requirement to collect many histopathological tissues from large numbers of animals. In these cases it is recommended that samples are sent to the laboratory at regular intervals to avoid unnecessary delays in blood smear preparation and subsequent analysis.

Samples collected from the abdominal aorta of rodents at post mortem risk tissue fluid contamination increasing the potential for platelet clumping, inducing platelets to degranulate and/or clump, activating the coagulation cascade and diluting the sample. Cells on a peripheral blood smear may distort due to differing protein concentrations and pH of tissue fluid, compared to peripheral blood. Delays in obtaining samples due to removal of other organs may compromise the quality of the sample.

Water-ice (used in organ preservation/preparation, e.g. rapid cooling of gel in lungs for histological examination of expanded alveoli), may induce partial freezing of cells in the underlying abdominal aorta, potentially causing hemolysis and leaving a mixture of spherocytes and "ghost" red cells in peripheral blood smears.

Sample transport and storage

Samples must be transported to the laboratory with minimal delay to minimise the potential for artifact

formation. Opinions vary on ideal transport and storage conditions for routine hematology samples[6], making it more relevant that appropriate procedures are established by the individual laboratory.

It may be that samples from different species require different transport and storage conditions; for example we have found that human samples are more reliable transported and stored at room temperature, whereas rodent samples are best maintained refrigerated or on cold blocks (<8°C) (unpublished data). Care must be taken to ensure that samples are not accidentally frozen, for example by keeping cold blocks frozen instead of refrigerated.

Transport delays and inappropriate storage (increased temperature) of rodent samples before analysis may induce rapid utilisation of intracellular adenosine tri-phosphate (ATP), breakdown of red cell energy reserves and rapid changes in red cell morphology (e.g. formation of burr cells/crenation[7]).

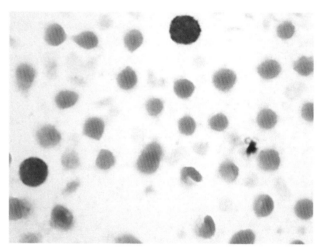

Photo 8.1 Spherocytes, large platelets and ghost red cells/cellular debris following partial freezing of a rat sample. Note: background staining of free hemoglobin (×1200).

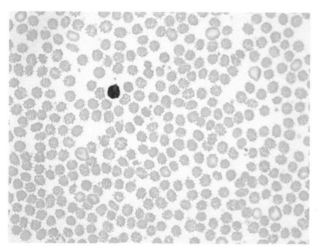

Photo 8.3 Crenated/burr cells in rat blood stored ambiently for 24 hours (×1200).

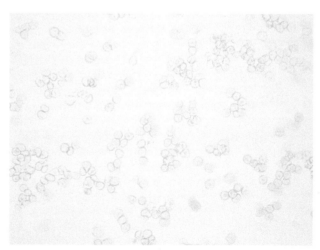

Photo 8.2 RBC ghosts created in a rat sample transported on a frozen cold block (×1000).

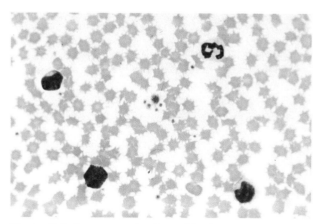

Photo 8.4 Severe crenation in pig blood stored ambiently for 24 hours (×1000).

Anticoagulant

High ratios of EDTA:blood will distort cells through osmotic effects causing red cell crenation and lowered mean corpuscular volume (MCV) (effectively increasing intracellular hemoglobin), producing small contracted cells on a blood smear. White cell identification may be difficult due to contracted cytoplasm and dark nuclei.

Conversely, too little anticoagulant will lead to activation of the sample, platelet degranulation, clumping/aggregation, coagulation cascade activation and, eventually, visible fibrin. Some species' platelets (e.g. cat, rabbit, pig, horse) aggregate easily presenting a dilemma on whether to report the platelet count (actual value or "at least"), red/white cell parameters only, the whole blood count (with/without a caveat to say the platelet count may not be accurate/reliable) or nothing at all (sample clotted). Spontaneous aggregation may be observed in samples from otherwise healthy cats, pigs and horses, particularly in samples collected into EDTA[8].

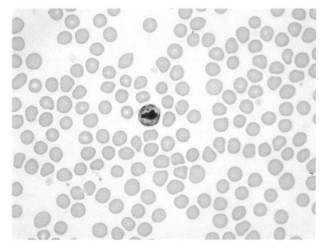

Photo 8.7 Concentrated EDTA effect on a white cell (×1000).

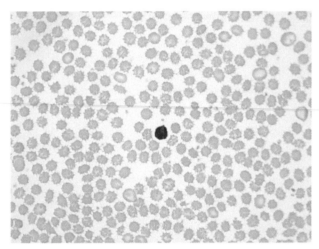

Photo 8.5 Crenated/burr cells in rat blood stored ambiently for 6 hours (×500).

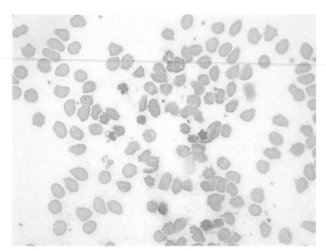

Photo 8.8 Concentrated EDTA effect on rat red cells (×1000).

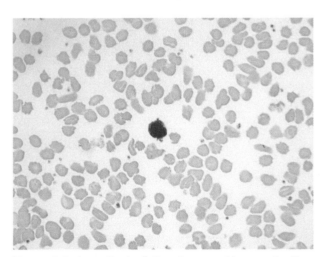

Photo 8.6 Generalised cell distortion caused by osmotic effects in rat blood (×1000).

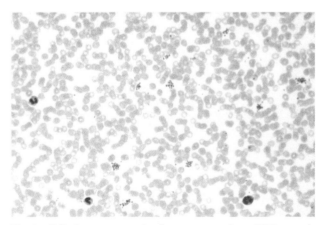

Photo 8.9 Spontaneous platelet aggregates in an EDTA sample from a healthy cat (×500).

Storage artifacts

Cells start to deteriorate on removal from the circulation; EDTA prevents the sample clotting and stabilises cell membranes[9], slowing cell degradation for a few days dependent on species and storage conditions. Normal morphology is preserved for approximately 5 hours at 4°C[10].

Erythrocytes of some rodent species change shape on storage[11] after approximately 6 hours due to factors such as pH change, effect of storage in glass tubes and/or slow drying of the blood smear. Hemoglobin crystals may also form.

Treatment with drugs, such as furosemide, amphiphilic agents, doxorubicin, phenyl hydrazine, and path-

ological causes, such as liver disease, lymphosarcoma, uremia, glomerulonephritis and metabolic diseases (e.g. electrolyte depletion in horses with hyponatremia and hypochloridemia), may lead to extracellular fluid loss and dehydration, causing artifactual crenation/echinocytes/burr cells. Formation of numerous short, regular, projections on the cell surface produces cellular enlargement affecting calculated parameters such as mean cell hemoglobin concentration (MCHC).

Echinocytes are common in normal healthy rodents and in unwell cats and dogs. They are often unreported as they are usually artifacts, or may indicate a non-specific abnormality, making it difficult to distinguish "real" from artifactual causes in the absence of other data.

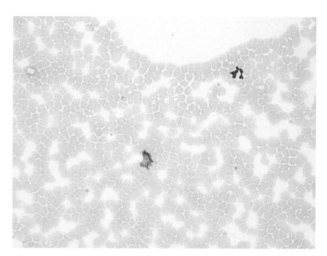

Photo 8.10 Rat peripheral blood dried slowly in a damp atmosphere (×500).

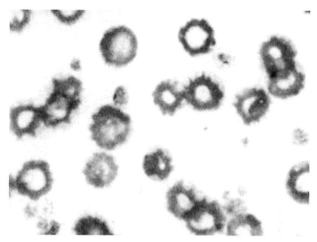

Photo 8.12 Echinocytes in the blood smear of a basenji dog with pyruvate kinase deficiency. Note polychromatophilic erythrocytes indicating erythroid regeneration (Wright–Leishman stain) (×1000).

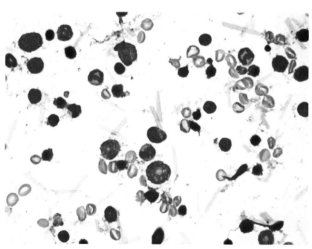

Photo 8.11 Rat bone marrow dried slowly in a very cold and damp atmosphere (×500).

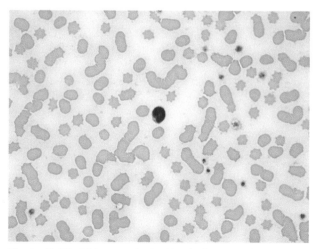

Photo 8.13 Echinocytes in the blood of a cat with peritonitis, possibly an artifact of blood smear preparation (Wright–Leishman stain). Note excessive rouleaux (×500).

Common artifacts in stored EDTA blood samples are macrocytosis[12] and distributional abnormalities, e.g. nucleated cells carried to the tail of the smear[13] due to poor mixing following overnight storage or due to increased adherence of abnormal cells.

Following storage at room temperature for a few days, white cells may develop irregular outlines or disintegrate entirely on spreading a blood film forming "smear cells", leading to an apparent reduced white cell count and/or inaccurate differential. Polymorphonuclear nuclei become dense, homogeneous and round (pyknotic), and may degenerate (necrobiotic), lobulate and fragment (karyolysis/apoptosis). Cytoplasmic vacuolation may occur as soon as 1 hour after collection[14].

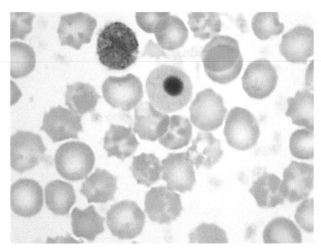

Photo 8.16 Degenerative changes in a hamster neutrophil and monocyte after storage at 4°C for 2 days (×1200).

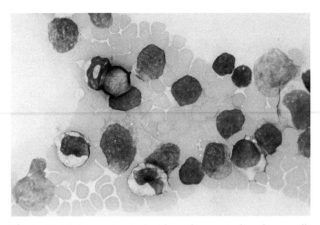

Photo 8.14 Mouse treated with methotrexate: lymphoma cells carried to the tail of the smear (×1000).

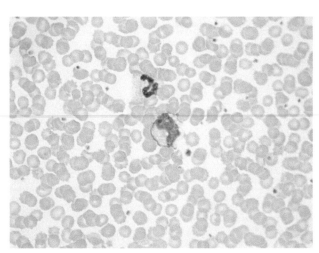

Photo 8.17 Monocytes accumulate vacuoles within 1 hour of collection (×1000).

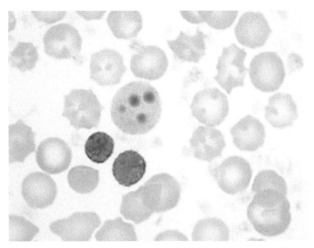

Photo 8.15 Degenerative changes in hamster neutrophil and lymphocytes after storage at 4°C for 2 days (×1200).

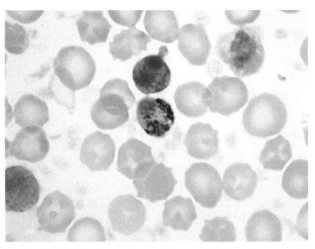

Photo 8.18 Numbers of pseudo-basophils in rodent samples increase following overnight storage (×1200).

Blood smear preparation

Preparation of a good quality blood smear is more than adequately documented in other publications[15,16] and is equally applicable to animal work.

Slow air drying of a smear in high humidity, or contamination of the fixative with water, will lead to red cells absorbing excess water producing spherocytes. Normal leukocytes may shrink and lymphocytes may exhibit a "hairy" appearance. Smear cells may be produced and appear as eosinophilic amorphous material, or bare nuclei.

Platelets may swell and appear pale when stained with Romanowsky stains and, when overlying red cells, may appear to be Howell–Jolly bodies; careful examination is necessary to avoid misinterpretation.

If platelets are activated during the collection process (not obvious on a *fresh* blood smear), the

blood clotting process may still proceed in the presence of anticoagulant and at cool temperatures, leading to aggregated platelets on a *subsequent* smear. Less commonly platelet satellitism may occur which will lead to erroneous platelet counts. "Pseudo-eosinophils" (due to platelet clumping) occur in mice following overnight sample storage leading to inaccurate automated differentials.

Stain precipitate

Dark purple granules of precipitated stain may be distributed in patches or scattered across large areas of a smear, and must be distinguished from bacteria or red cell parasites.

Stain precipitate in feline blood smears could be mistaken for erythroparasites, e.g. *Haemobartonella felis*, which are seen as individual small cocci, chains, rods and occasional "ring" forms. Even with the benefit of special stains, e.g. May–Grünwald Giemsa, these are notoriously difficult to identify. The main difficulties are: low parasitemias; the presence of stain precipitate; and refractile bodies. Stain precipitate will be present both on and in the spaces between RBCs. Refractile bodies, unlike parasites, tend to be associated with RBCs, show refractivity when focusing and vary more in size[17].

Occasionally cells may be observed that have an amusing appearance and, although of no particular diagnostic or toxicological relevance, still bring a smile to the face.

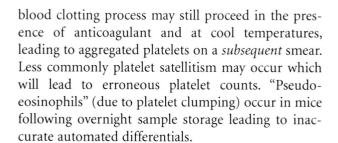

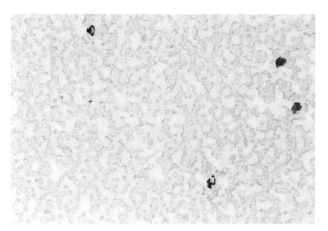

Photo 8.19 Poor methanol fixation of a dog blood smear (×1000).

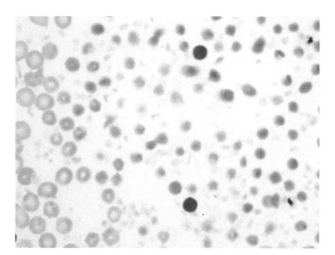

Photo 8.20 Spherocytes induced by excess water absorption during smear preparation (×500).

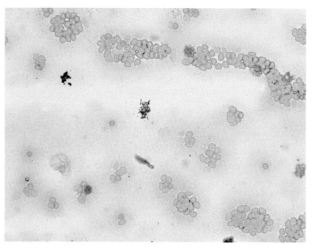

Photo 8.21 Stain deposit (modified Wright) on a rat smear (×1000).

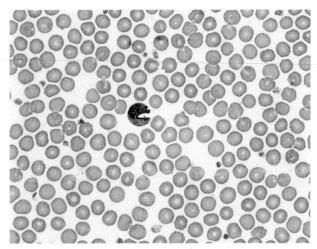

Photo 8.22 A "Pacman" cell – a genuine photograph (×1000).

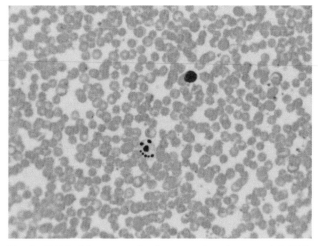

Photo 8.24 A "snowman" cell – a genuine photograph (×500).

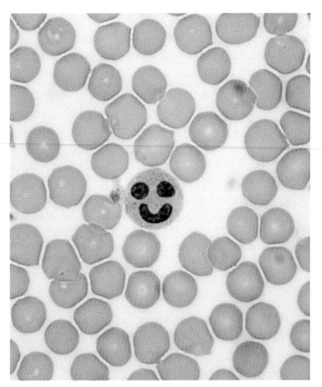

Photo 8.23 "Smiley" – a genuine photograph with the nuclear bridges removed using Photo-enhancing software (×1200).

References

1. Encarta World English Dictionary. http://uk.encarta. msn.com/encnet/features/dictionary/Dictionary Results.aspx?lextype=3&search=artefact
2. Schwabenbauer C (1991). Influence of the blood sampling site on some haematological and clinical chemical parameters in Sprague-Dawley rats. *Comp Haematol Int* 1: 112–116.
3. Rovira S, Munoz A, Benito M (2007). Hematologic and biochemical changes during canine agility competitions. *Vet Clin Pathol* 36(1): 30–35.
4. Matsuzawa T, Sakazume M (1994). Effects of fasting on haematology and clinical chemistry values in the rat and dog. *Comp Haematol Int* 4: 152–156.
5. Nemzek JA, Bolgos GL, Williams BA, Remick DG (2001). Differences in normal values for murine white blood cell counts and other haematological parameters based on sampling site. *Inflamm Res* 50(10): 523–527.
6. Hayashi Y, Matsuzawa T, *et al.* (1995) Effects on haematology parameters during cold storage and cold transport of rat and dog blood samples. *Comp Haematol Int* 5: 251–255.
7. Fox JG (2007). *The Rat in Biomedical Research.* New York: Academic Press.
8. Gresele P, Page C, Fuster V, Vermylen J (2002). Platelets in thrombotic and non-thrombotic disorders. In: *Pathophysiology, Pharmacology and Therapeutics.* Cambridge: Cambridge University Press, 348.
9. www.vetstreamlapis.co.uk/htmlroot/Tables/lab60015. htm
10. Patel N (2009). Why is EDTA the anticoagulant of choice for hematology use? *Tech Talk* 7(1).
11. Bain B (2001). *Blood Cells – A Practical Guide.* Oxford: Blackwell Publishing.
12. www.lvlabs.co.uk/pdf/library/DAVNHaematologyLN. pdf
13. Red cell morphology in health and disease. www.med. univ-angers.fr/discipline/lab_hema/morphogrweb/ webmorphohematie.html
14. Koepke JA (1991). *Practical Laboratory Haematology.* New York: Churchill Livingstone.
15. Pierre RV (2002). Interpretation of the peripheral blood film. *Clin Lab Med* (22)1: 25–61.
16. Lewis SM, Bain BJ, Bates I (2010). *Dacie and Lewis Practical Haematology (10th edn).* Edinburgh: Churchill Livingstone.
17. www.lvlabs.co.uk/pdf/library/AnaemiaLN.pdf

9

Bone marrow

Geoff Brown

Introduction

Bone marrow evaluation requires collection of good quality samples if subsequent analyses are to be of diagnostic value. Traditionally, bone marrow examination has been approached from two directions – production of a smear from an aspirate; and a histological section from a trephine biopsy, or sample of bone removed at post mortem. Both give valuable information on marrow activity, but are essentially complementary: a smear does not give an accurate picture of total cellularity or of structural architecture, whereas histological preparations obscure many important details necessary for proper classification of cell maturation. Without such classification, subsequent statistical analysis, such as the calculation of myeloid and erythroid left shift indices[1], becomes impossible. For complete analysis, both types of preparation should be examined[2,3].

Clotting and cell degeneration in marrow occur rapidly after death or resection; rapid sampling and smear preparation are essential if accurate interpretation is to be made either in a clinical situation or at the end of a toxicity study. Seybold et al.[4] refer to the short coagulation time of bone marrow, whilst Valli et al.[5] put the clotting time after death at only 2–3 minutes. Tyler et al.[6] comment on the rapid degeneration of the marrow, and recommend that samples be taken within 30 minutes of death. These changes may be slowed by storing the material at 4°C either as discrete bone removed on death[7] or as a suspension on albumin[8].

Clearly, then, there is an advantage in taking marrow samples from a live animal, but in a drug safety testing situation where regulatory authorities are increasingly reluctant to licence such procedures, this is not always possible. Alternatively, samples should be taken immediately after death in order to minimise clotting and degenerative changes.

Review of marrow sampling techniques

From the live animal

Many methods and variations have been published for the aspiration of marrow from larger animals (e.g. cats, dogs, horses), although all use an appropriate intramedullary needle (e.g. Rosenthal, Gimson, etc.) introduced into the marrow cavity by a twisting motion with hand pressure, followed by aspiration under vacuum using a 10–30 mL syringe. Local anesthetic at the site of operation is usually sufficient[2,4,9], but some authors recommend a general anesthetic, particularly with cats[10].

Many aspiration sites have been used, with the iliac crest, femur, humerus and sternum being the most common. Choice of site depends on operator preference since it is claimed that (the shafts of long bones in adults excepted) marrow activity is generally homogeneous throughout the body[3,11]. Most authors do not

Atlas of Comparative Diagnostic and Experimental Hematology, Second Edition. Clifford Smith, Alfred Jarecki.
© 2011 Blackwell Publishing Ltd. Published 2011 by Blackwell Publishing Ltd.

use anticoagulants for the procedure, but EDTA is recommended where necessary, e.g. where a large number of smears is required[12].

For smaller animals, most published methods are concerned with rats, although these techniques have been successfully used with guinea pigs, hamsters, young rabbits and even mice. Some use specially designed or modified needles[13,14,15], whilst others use a dentist's drill or equivalent to assist in piercing the bone[16]. In the latter method final aspiration of the marrow is achieved using a glass capillary tube or pipette. The most commonly used site for aspiration in small animals is the femur, although the iliac crest[14] and the tibia[16] have also been used. All of these methods can, with care, be performed on a recovery basis.

Aspiration from live animals, whether achieved by natural flow into a capillary (e.g. rats), or by suction using a 10 or 20 mL syringe, will only yield a small quantity of marrow, i.e. that marrow available in the immediate vicinity of the puncture. Once this is obtained, further aspiration will only be of blood, and excessive dilution of the samples with blood will make the resultant smears uninterpretable. Many authors stress "small volumes" or "a few drops"[2,6,9], whilst others specify maximum volumes, e.g. 200–300 µL in horses[17] or 5 µL in rats[5]. These figures are broadly in line with the author's recommendations of up to 250 µL in larger animals (dogs and primates) and 3 µL in rats.

Post mortem

At post mortem, irrespective of its size, marrow is normally obtained by exposing or removing a bone, opening it by splitting or cutting, and removing a small quantity of marrow with forceps[7], a small paintbrush[18] or some other appropriate implement (e.g. scalpel blade). If this is done within 2–3 minutes of death, the subsequent marrow sample can be spread readily, but at a longer time after death than this, some means of freeing the cells from the resultant clot is required.

Recommended methods for marrow sampling

From the live animal

It should be stressed that the methods referred to above will work well under optimum conditions, i.e. experienced operators using the right equipment, and having plenty of time to attend to every detail – conditions which are not always met in a busy post-mortem room. As a result, samples are best taken from the live animal prior to death, using techniques that are as rapid and simple as possible, consistent with good readable samples.

The techniques described below meet these requirements and achieve a high success rate. Both methods can, with care, be performed on a recovery basis, making it possible to take multiple samples during the course of a study. However, to ensure complete recovery, samples should not be taken from the same site more frequently than every 10–14 days. For the occasional sample that does not reach the required standard (usually due to excessive blood contamination), a section of an appropriate bone should always be available.

For larger animals (dogs, primates, pigs, calves, sheep, rabbits, etc.), the following method is very successful. For dogs, primates and rabbits the operation can easily be performed under local anesthetic (e.g. lidocaine hydrochloride), but for other species a general anesthetic is normally used (e.g. pentobarbital).

Following the administration of anesthetic, the animal is placed on its back; when a local anesthetic is used the animal should be reclined against an experienced handler. The area over the sternum is shaved and swabbed with an appropriate sterilising agent. A Gimson's intramedullary needle is recommended which is obtainable in various lengths below the fixed guard or variations may be purchased with an adjustable guard. For most species, a working length of 18–32 mm is sufficient.

The needle is pushed through the skin and inserted into the sternum using a twisting motion and hand pressure. When the cavity is entered a slight "give" will be felt, and the needle will move laterally, but remain firm in the bone. The handle, together with the stillette, is removed, and a 10–20 mL syringe is attached to the needle. Full vacuum is applied which is released as soon as marrow begins to flow into the syringe, to ensure that the maximum volume of 250 µL is not exceeded.

The syringe and needle are withdrawn together and direct pressure is applied to the puncture wound for 1–2 minutes. Two smears are made direct from the needle, in the same way as blood smears[19]. Additional smears may be prepared, or the remainder placed into EDTA for the performance of total cell count, if required. In the author's experience, however, total nucleated cell counts by this method are of limited value, since dilution with blood cannot be assessed – a histological section of a rib or femur, etc., will indicate total cellularity more accurately. Alternatively, the remainder may be placed into a suitable medium for subsequent evaluation using flow cytometry methods.

For small animals (rats, guinea pigs, hamsters), the following method is particularly useful. It can also be successfully applied to rabbits, although sternal puncture is more convenient with this species. Success with mice has been limited – for these animals, a post-mortem procedure is more likely to give satisfactory results.

A general anesthetic (e.g. pentobarbital) is administered, and the animal placed on its back. One hind-limb is extended and held in place by applying pressure at the top of the thigh between the thumb and fore-finger. An incision is made in the skin along the line of the tibia, a second incision being made along the same line to separate the muscle capsule: this will allow for easy retraction of the muscles without causing undue damage. A hole is drilled in the top of the exposed tibia using a hand-held drill and a dentist's burr. The hole should be marginally bigger than the capillary being used to collect the marrow, and drilling is facilitated if it is performed at the relatively flat area close to the head of the bone.

As with larger animals, a slight "give" will be felt when the drill enters the bone cavity. The drill is removed, and a glass capillary inserted into the hole. Pressure at the top of the thigh is relaxed, and marrow will flow into the capillary: Use of a graduated capillary is recommended to ensure that the maximum volume of 3 μL is not exceeded. Smears are made directly from the capillary. In normal toxicological practice the animal is sacrificed without recovery but if care has been taken with this operation rapid recovery is possible by sealing the hole in the bone with beeswax, and closing the incision with a clip[16].

Post mortem

Once an animal is dead, irrespective of size/species, the whole or part of a bone is removed, and the marrow extracted from it. The method of extraction will depend on how long the animal has been dead: as stated previously, if this procedure is carried out within 2–3 minutes of death, the marrow will not have clotted, and this will be of great assistance in making a good smear.

In a toxicological post-mortem room the following method will give consistently good results. Following the death of an animal a bone should be immediately removed and passed to a trained assistant. The bone will normally be the femur in rats and mice, and either the sternum or a rib in larger animals.

The bone is stripped of contaminating tissue (muscle, membranes etc.) and then split using a pair of bone cutters. A small paintbrush, moistened with an appropriate medium (autologous serum or plasma, or bovine albumin at a concentration of between 1 and 10%), is inserted into the exposed cavity and cells removed. A series of "streaks" of the cellular/medium mixture is then painted on to a glass slide. When this is complete, the paintbrush is cleaned with isotonic saline before collecting the next sample.

When using this method it is important to use fresh medium regularly in order to avoid bacterial contamination, which in extreme cases could make the compilation of a myelogram impossible.

An alternative method, which involves storing removed bones at 4°C until further manipulation, is useful[7]. Following the storage period, which in practise can be up to 3 hours, the bones are stripped and the marrow cavity is opened as described above, and a portion of the marrow (now clotted) removed using a pair of forceps. This portion is gently squeezed to free the cells from the clot, and mixed with a small amount of 5% albumin prior to making a smear. It is important not to use too much albumin (the volume of albumin in the albumin–marrow mixture should be 50% or less), as this will result in a blue-staining background[8] and/or condensation of some cellular elements, both of which will make subsequent cellular identification difficult or impossible. Care must also be taken to ensure that the mixing process is not too violent as this will cause undue destruction of some cells, more primitive cells are likely to suffer most[20].

Where larger samples of marrow are required (for example when carrying out analysis by flow cytometry), removal of the total marrow from the femur of rodents may be necessary. This may be accomplished by removing one or both femurs immediately after death, and stripping away contaminating tissue as described above, after which the femoral head and the distal epiphysis of each femur are removed using an electric saw.

Bone marrow tissue is gently flushed out and a single cell suspension is then prepared by drawing the marrow suspension gently back and forth through the needle prior to further manipulation[21].

Preparation and staining of smears

Having obtained a suitable sample, making the smear is of prime importance: many methods have been published, some requiring considerable manipulation. For production of normal smears, minimum manipulation should be used to prevent cell damage and destruction, which, as stated earlier, tends to occur most often in the more primitive cells. With the possibility of having to prepare several hundred smears at the end of a long-term carcinogenicity study, the spreading of smears directly from the needle or capillary, as described above for live animals, meets both the need for speed and minimal handling.

Such methods have been described by several authors[13,15,17], and although these preparations contain variable amounts of blood, this can be kept to a minimum by limiting the sample size. Indeed, the presence of mature red cells appears to offer some protection to nucleated cells, and the resultant cellular detail is well worth the relative inability to assess total cellularity, which in any case is better assessed by histological section.

Traditional methods of expressing a marrow aspirate on to an inclined glass slide or petri dish where marrow particles will stick (allowing excess blood to drain), followed frequently by a squash preparation, are extremely time consuming and therefore only practical when preparing single or few samples[4,6,9].

For samples removed immediately after death the "paintbrush" method also includes the method of smear preparation as part of the procedure, as does the method described for the removal of marrow from bones stored for up to 3 hours at 4°C.

Other methods for preparing smears from postmortem samples include the "contact" method, in which a portion of marrow is dragged across a slide leaving a trail of cells adhering to it and "rolling" the clotted marrow along the length of the slide by persistently lifting the clot up at the back, using a needle or similar object[6]. These latter methods can yield extremely good results, but in the author's experience cannot always be guaranteed.

Samples intended for flow cytometric analysis must, by definition, be subject to special preparative techniques, and during the course of these manipulations it is possible to prepare a monolayer film of the marrow cells using the Cytospin system (Shandon,

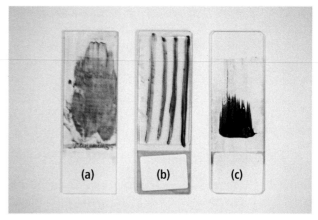

Photo 9.1 Macroscopic appearance of stained smears produced by: (a) squash method; (b) streak method; (c) spread method.

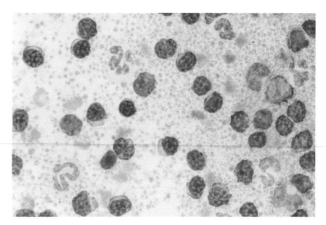

Photo 9.2 Cytospin preparation showing morphology of platelets and lymphoblasts (×1000).

England). The bone marrow cell suspension obtained as described above is filtered through a 100 μL filter device, underlayed with 1 mL fetal calf serum and centrifuged at 300 g for 5 minutes at 4°C. The supernatant containing most of the fat cells is discarded, and the cellular pellet re-suspended in cold PBS containing 5% bovine serum albumin. After counting the nucleated cells in the suspension and adjusting the total to ~100 cells/mL with PBS, but prior to incubation with appropriate monoclonal antibodies, aliquots may be taken for slide preparation using the Cytospin[21]; such preparations are frequently used to compare or confirm changes seen in the flow cytometric results.

A similar method may also be used to make Cytospin preparations alone. Although these films are normally of excellent quality, the time taken for their production is excessive and does not easily fit with the time available for routine terminal assays at the end of a toxicological study.

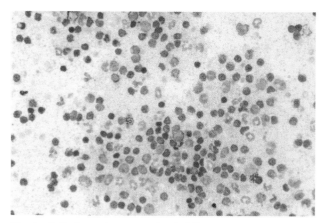

Photo 9.3 Cytospin preparation (×20).

Once made, smears should be air-dried and fixed in methanol for 20 minutes. Any Romanowsky stain may be used for routine evaluation (Leishman, May–Grünwald Giemsa, modified Wright's, etc.), but for optimum results staining times should be considerably increased over that normally used for blood smears (up to twice as long). This appears to be critical for samples removed at post mortem.

Unstained smears may be air-dried overnight prior to fixing in formalin vapor, after which various cytochemical stains may be applied[7,12].

Evaluation

An initial scan should be made of the stained marrow smear under a relatively low-power objective (×20 or ×40). At this magnification assessment of cellularity, or of the possibility of excessive blood contamination, may be made. In smears where very few nucleated cells are present, and especially where marrow aplasia is suspected from other findings, the difference between true aplasia and blood contamination must be appreciated. In true aplasia non-myeloid cells (e.g. lymphocytes, plasma cells) will predominate with only an occasional precursor cell, whereas excessive blood contamination will result in a smear containing predominately mature cells of all types, together with many precursors.

At this initial scan it is also possible to identify cells arranged in unusual patterns (e.g. rosetting, agglutination, excessive rouleaux of mature red cells), and to locate areas of relatively high nucleated cell concentrations. Where such concentrations exist the detailed count should be made in this area. If nucleated cells appear in a more or less even distribution across the smear, detailed counts should be made across the film

at a point where cells are sufficiently separated to allow for positive identification. In such cases at least 20% of the cells should be counted close to the edge or tail of the smear to take account of any possible uneven distribution of the various cell types.

Full myelograms are made using a high-power objective (×100), and a minimum of 500 cells should be counted. Cells are traditionally classified into the various stages of maturation for myeloid and erythroid cells. At completion of the count the myeloid : erythroid (M : E) ratio is calculated by dividing the total number of myeloid cells counted by the total number of erythroid cells counted[22].

Where an abnormal result has been obtained or is suspected, interpretation is often made easier by the calculation of the myeloid and erythroid left shift indices (M-LSI, E-LSI). This is done by dividing the total number of myeloblasts, promyelocytes, myelocytes, metamyelocytes and band forms by the total number of neutrophils, eosinophils and basophils for the M-LSI; and by dividing the total number of pro-erythroblasts and early normoblasts by the total number of intermediate and late normoblasts[1] for the E-LSI.

In addition to the counts, differences in cell morphology, the appearance of unusual cell patterns, or any other observed abnormality which could aid interpretation should be noted and included in the final report.

As a quicker alternative to a full myelogram a straightforward calculation of the M : E ratio may be performed by counting total myeloid cells, erythroid cells and others, without categorising them further. A minimum of 200 cells should be counted, and the calculation made as described above.

Interpretation

As with any clinical pathology parameter, interpretation of bone marrow data should never be made in isolation. Clinical signs, the results of hematological and clinical chemistry assays, post-mortem findings and, where appropriate, histopathological findings must all be taken into account.

This is particularly important when analysing samples taken at the time of, or close to the onset of, an acute reaction. Acute reactions frequently lead to a series of dynamic changes in the marrow in response to the insult. For example, a sudden intravascular hemolytic crisis will lead to marked increase in erythropoesis, but this may take several hours to become readily apparent in the marrow and samples taken too close to the onset of such a crisis may show little or no change, possibly giving the impression that the marrow is unaffected by the insult.

If a full myelogram has been performed, the E-LSI will show such changes earlier than the M : E ratio, but even this change may be subject to a slight delay; in such cases it is useful to examine a further sample of marrow 24 hours later. In the case of toxicity studies this should be on other animals where clinical signs suggest a greater time lapse from the initial crisis or on animals from a lower dose group where any effects are likely to take longer to become established giving information on marrow changes, if any, at a stage preceding the crisis. Such further evaluations frequently show a pattern of response, consequently making diagnosis easier. Similarly, cytotoxic compounds may well induce morphological changes in cells, particularly on early forms.

In conclusion, the full and proper evaluation of bone marrow samples will provide many clues to the accurate diagnosis of many hematological conditions, and may well be predictive of further changes to come.

References

1. Brown G (1991). The left shift index: a useful guide to the interpretation of bone marrow data. *Comp Haematol Int* 1(2): 106–111.
2. Grindem CB (1989). Bone marrow biopsy and evaluation. *Vet Clin North Am* 19(4): 669–696.
3. Jacobs RM, Valli VEO (1988). Bone marrow biopsies: principles and perspectives of interpretation. *Sem Vet Med Surg* 3: 176.
4. Seybold IM, Goldston RT, Wilkes RD (1980). The clinical pathology laboratory. Examination of the bone marrow. *Vet Med Small Anim Clin* 75(10): 1517–1521.
5. Jones TC, Ward JM, Mohr U, Hunt RD (eds) (1994). Evaluation of blood and bone marrow in the rat. In: *Monograph of the Pathology of Laboratory Animals – Haemopoietic System* 86(3): 187–212.
6. Tyler RD, Cowell RL, Meinkoth JH (1999). Bone marrow. In: Cowell RL, Tyler RD, Meinkoth JH (eds) *Diagnostic Cytology of the Dog and Cat (2nd edn)*. St Louis: Mosby, 284–304.
7. Andrews CM (1991). The preparation of bone marrow smears from femurs obtained at autopsy. *Comp Haematol Int* 1(4): 229–232.
8. Berenbaum MC (1956). The use of bovine albumin the preparation of marrow and blood films. *J Clin Pathol* 9: 381–383.
9. Duncan JR, Prasse KW (1976). Clinical examination of bone marrow. *Vet Clin North Am* 6(4): 597–608.
10. Connor GH, Gupta BN, Krehbiel JD (1971). A technique for bone marrow biopsy in the cat. *J Am Vet Med Assoc* 158(10): 1702–1705.
11. Penny RHC, Carlisle CH (1970). The bone marrow biopsy of the dog: a comparative study of biopsy material obtained from the iliac crest, rib and sternum. *J Small Anim Pract* 11: 727–734.
12. Relford RL (1991). The steps in performing a bone marrow aspiration and core biopsy. *Vet Med* 86(7): 670–688.
13. Note S, Tsunematsu T, Ueno K, Tanaka A, Inagaki H, Yokoyama N, Ito T, Shinobe N, Wakizaka N, Kumura C (1961). Studies of rat bone marrow by means of a new puncture method. *Acta Haematol Jpn* 24: 16–21.
14. Brodsky SG, Arsenault A (1976). A rapid method for bone marrow aspiration in the rat. *Lab Anim Sci* 26(5): 826 827.
15. Archer RK, Riley J, Gwilliam RVE (1981). Aspiration of bone marrow from laboratory rats. *Br J Haematol* 48: 165–166.
16. Desaga JF, Parwaresch MR (1970). A new method for sequential detection of bone marrow cells in small laboratory animals. *Blut* 21: 176–179.
17. Franken P, Wensing TH, Schotman AJH (1982). The bone marrow of the horse: 1. The techniques of sampling, examination and values of normal warm-blooded horses. *Zbl Vet Med* A29: 16–22.
18. Albanese R, Middleton BJ (1987). The assessment of micronucleated polychromatic erythrocytes in rat bone marrow. *Mutat Res* 182(6): 323–332.
19. Dacie JV, Lewis SM (2010). *Practical Haematology (10th edn)*. Edinburgh: Churchill Livingstone.
20. Beck CC, Connor GH, Ross BH (1971). Serial bone marrow biopsies. *Vet Med Small Anim Clin* 66(9): 917–920.
21. Saad A, Palm M, Widell S, Reiland S (2000). Differential analysis of rat bone marrow by flow cytometry. *Comp Haematol Int* 10(2): 97–101.
22. Jain NC (1993). *Essentials of Veterinary Haematology*. Philadelphia: Lea and Febiger.

10

Comparative applications in flow cytometry

Alaa Saad

Flow cytometry is a technology for measuring optical and fluorescence characteristics of cells in a suspension of a heterogeneous mixture of cells. Today's flow cytometer was originally developed as a microscopic based device in the middle of the last century. At the same time, Wallace Coulter introduced the use of electrodes to measure the electric conductance of cells in a suspension through a tiny orifice. This lead to the introduction of the first commercial cell counters in 1960.

Commercial cytometers with increasing sensitivity, complexity, computerisation and practicality appeared during the late 1970s such as Cytofluorograph (Ortho), FACS-III and FACStarPLUS (Becton-Dickinson), Spectrum III (Ortho), EPICS (Coulter) etc. The need for a fair degree of expertise combined with the instrumentation costs and complexity, limited the early use of flow cytometry to research laboratories and specialised clinical institutes. Flow cytometry rapidly gained a wide range of clinical applications including the integration of flow cytometry techniques into routine hematology analysers.

Commercial availability of monoclonal antibodies initially limited the use of flow cytometry in various animal species. However, the utilisation of flow cytometry in veterinary research and clinical studies has increased, including applications in hematology, immunology, sperm quality and sorting, chromosome karyotyping and dairy science.

The basic components of a flow cytometer are a laser light source, a fluidic sample chamber (flow cell) and optical assembly. The cells are hydro-dynamically focused in a sheath fluid before intersecting an optimally focused laser. Scattered and emitted light is collected by a series of filters and dichroic mirrors that isolate particular wavelength bands and then converted to digital electrical pulses by photomultiplier tubes (PMT) so that they may be stored for later display and computer analysis. The resulting information is usually displayed in one-parameter histogram or two dimensional dot-plot formats.

Some light is scattered at very small angles (3–12°) and this is referred to as forward angle light scatter (FSC), which is directly related to the diameter of the cell and will therefore represent the relative size of the cell. Light that is scattered at larger angles (90°) is proportional to the magnitude of cellular granularity or internal complexity, and this is referred to as right angle or side scatter (SSC). Size and density are very important criteria used extensively in hematology analysers to distinguish between different lineages of blood cells.

If the cells are tagged with specific fluorescent marker(s), the fluorescent molecules can be excited to an elevated energy state by laser light, and emit light energy at a higher wavelength. The fluorescence emissions at different wavelengths are also detected 90° to the incident laser beam with PMTs. The use of several

Atlas of Comparative Diagnostic and Experimental Hematology, Second Edition. Clifford Smith, Alfred Jarecki.
© 2011 Blackwell Publishing Ltd. Published 2011 by Blackwell Publishing Ltd.

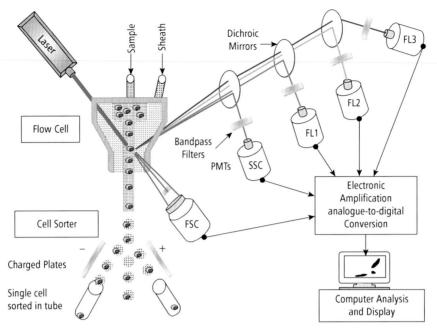

Figure 10.1 Schematic drawing of basic flow cytometry.

flurochromes (similar excitation wavelength and different emission wavelengths) allows several cell properties to be measured simultaneously. The detection limit is as low as 100 fluorescent molecules per cell. The most important feature of flow cytometry is the rapid (at rates of 1 000 to 30 000 cells/second) correlated measurements of multiple properties of a single cell.

Application of flow cytometry in comparative hematology

Hematology analysers

Although several flow cytometry based "five-part differential" hematology analysers commercially exist in the market, few of them have the software to analyse the peripheral blood of animal species. Brief descriptions of the most common analysers with integrated veterinary application are given below.

ADVIA® 120 and ADVIA® 2120

Leukocytes are classified by the ADVIA instruments (Siemens Medical Solutions Diagnostics) based on the level of myeloperoxidase content, following cytochemical staining with 4-chloro-1-naphthol in the presence of hydrogen peroxide, and cell size. The absorbance signal (peroxidase staining) and the forward light-scattering signal (cell size) of each blood

cell are measured in the PEROX channel. Normal neutrophils and eosinophils possess significant levels of peroxidase activity, monocytes contain lower amounts of peroxidase, while lymphocytes, basophils and large unstained cells contain no granules with peroxidase enzyme activity.

In the BASO channel, a reagent containing a combination of acid and surfactant strips the cytoplasm of leukocytes and lyses red blood cells. The sample is then analysed by two-angle laser light scattering detection using a laser diode. Leukocytes are categorised as mononuclear or polymorphonuclear cells based on the shape and complexity of their nuclei. Intact basophils, which are particularly resistant to lysis by the reagent, can be easily distinguished from the smaller cell nuclei.

Both red blood cells and platelets are analysed in the BASO channel after appropriate dilution of the blood with a reagent that isovolumetrically spheres and lightly fixes the red cells. Red cells and platelets are counted from the signals from a common detector with two different gain settings. The platelet signals are amplified considerably more than the RBC signals.

Reticulocytes are also analysed in the BASO channel following staining with a nucleic acid dye (oxazine 750) to stain cellular RNA and a reagent to isovolumetrically sphere erythroid cells. Low-angle laser light scatter, high-angle laser light scatter and absorption characteristics of all cells are measured. The absorp-

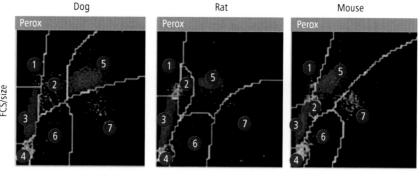

Figure 10.2 WBC differential analysis in the PEROX channel of an ADVIA analyser. 1, large unstained cells; 2, monocytes; 3, lymphocytes; 4, noise; 5, neutrophils; 6, platelet clumps; 7, eosinophils.

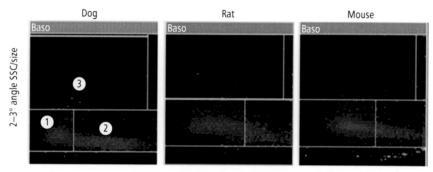

Figure 10.3 WBC differential analysis in the BASO channel of an ADVIA analyser. 1, mononuclear cells; 2, polymorphonuclear cells; 3, basophils.

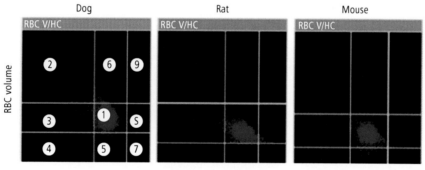

Figure 10.4 RBC cell-by-cell analysis in the BASO channel of an ADVIA analyser. 1, normochromic normocytic; 2, hypochromic macrocytic; 3, hypochromic normocytic; 4, hypochromic microcytic; 5, normochromic microcytic; 6, normochromic macrocytic; 7, hyperchromic microcytic; 8, hyperchromic microcytic; 9, hyperchromic macrocytic.

tion data are used to classify each cell as a reticulocyte or mature red blood cell based on its RNA content.

CellDyn 3500

The CellDyn 3500 hematology analyser (Abbott Diagnostics) employs dual technologies to provide the basis for a five-part white blood cell differential. Multiangle polarized scatter separation (MAPSS) provides

the primary white blood cell count and differential analysis, while the impedance channel provides additional information on the presence of fragile lymphocytes and hypotonically resistant red blood cells.

Sysmex XT-2000iv

Leukocyte differential analysis is performed on the Sysmex XT instrument using fluorescence flow

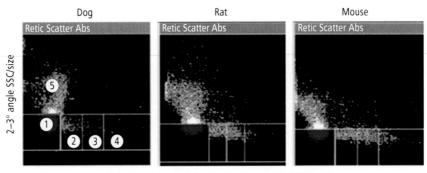

Light absorbance/Oxazine staining intensity/Cell Maturation

Figure 10.5 Retic/RBC cell-by-cell analysis in the BASO channel of an ADVIA analyser. 1, mature RBCs; reticulocytes with low (2), medium (3) and high (4) absorption; 5 , coincidence events.

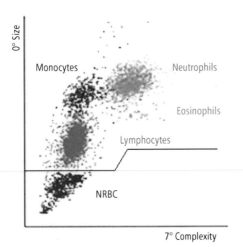

Figure 10.6 WBC differential analysis in the optical channel (WOC) of a CellDyn analyser.

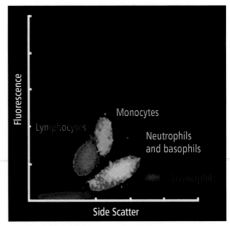

Figure 10.7 WBC differential analysis in the DIFF channel (fluorescence) of a Sysmex XT-2000iv analyser.

cytometry (FFC). A reagent containing a surfactant lyses red cells and platelets and permeabilises the membranes of white cells. A second reagent containing fluorescent dye specifically stains white cell nuclei as well as other cellular components. In the DIFF channel, the XT-series differentiates white cells into neutrophils and basophils together, eosinophils, monocytes and lymphocytes, and additionally determines immature granulocytes. Identification of basophils is performed in the WBC/Baso channel where all cells except for basophils are shrunk under the influence of the specific reagent.

HEMAVET® 950

The HEMAVET® 950 from Drew Scientific is specifically designed veterinary hematology analyser. HEMAVET® 950 uses species-specific diluting and patented focused-flow technology, and expectation maximisation software to perform five-part white blood cell differential in a wide range of animal species.

VetScan® HM5 Hematology

The VetScan HM5 (Abaxis Veterinary Diagnostics) uses a combination of chemical differentiation and impedance technology to provide a five-part white blood cell differential. The size of the pulse generated is directly proportional to the volume of each cell. This size discrimination, along with susceptibility to various lysing agents distinguishes the cell types and provides the basis for a five-part differential. In five-part differential mode only dog, cat and horse are included, while in the three-part differential mode, currently validated species are rat, rabbit, ferret, pig and cattle.

Bone marrow analysis

Several published methods describe the utilisation of flow cytometry for the analysis of bone marrow from different animal species. For rodents, Martin *et al.*[1] described a flow cytometric method based on membrane potential using 3,3′-dihexloxcarbocyanine iodide (DioC6) staining.

A combination of 2′,7′-dichlorofluorescein-diacetate staining (indirect myeloperoxidase staining) and monoclonal antibodies for lymphocyte subpopulations (OX52 for T-lymphocyte and OX4 for B-lymphocyte) was used by Criswell et al.[2] for the differential analysis of rat bone marrow.

Saad et al.[3] described a method for rat bone marrow differential using a combination of two monoclonal antibodies for the differential expression of leukocyte common antigen (CD45) and transferrin receptor (CD71). This was coupled with the side scatter for the cellular complexity nucleic acid staining with LDS-751 for the separation of nucleated cell from mature red blood cells.

A similar approach was used for rat bone marrow analysis (Saad et al. unpublished data). In addition, Schomaker et al.[4] described a method for rat bone marrow analysis using CD71 and scatter properties.

Weiss DJ (2004)[5] has used flow cytometry for dog bone marrow analysis based on cellular complexity and the expression of CD45. A similar approach but with the addition of LDS-751 staining was used by Saad et al. (unpublished data).

In addition, Saad et al. (unpublished data) used a combined CD45: FITC/LDS-751 method for dog bone marrow analysis with the newly introduced canine CD34 monoclonal antibody (progenitor/stem cell marker).

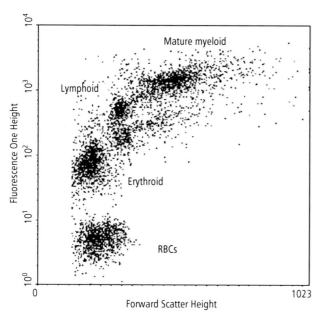

Figure 10.8 Rat bone marrow differential analysis using DiOC6 staining.

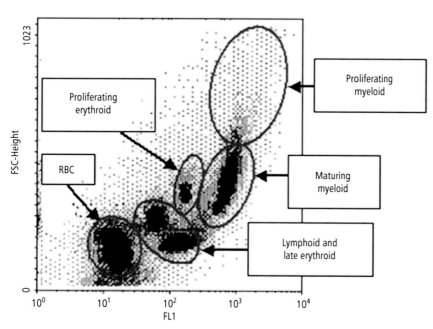

Figure 10.9 Rat bone marrow differential analysis using 2′,7′-dichlorofluorescein diacetate staining (indirect myeloperoxidase staining).

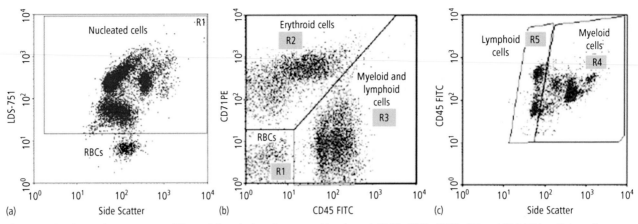

Figure 10.10 Rat bone marrow differential analysis using a combination of CD45: FITC, CD71: PE and LDS-751 staining. Cytogram C represents events in gate 3 of cytogram B.

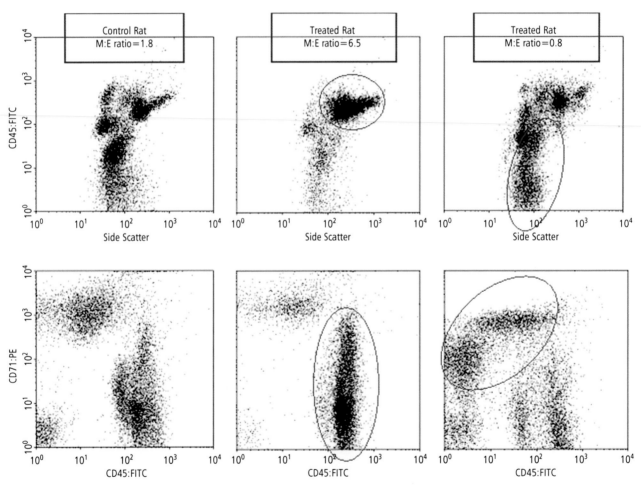

Figure 10.11 Rat bone marrow differential analysis of a control rat with an M : E ratio of 1.8 (left), a treated rat showing myeloid hyperplasia, a decrease in lymphoid and erythroid lineage, an M : E ratio of 6.5 (middle), and another treated rat showing an erythroid hyperplasia and M : E ratio of 0.8 (right).

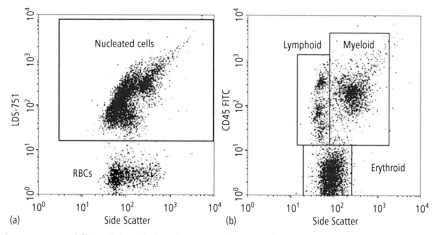

Figure 10.12 Dog bone marrow differential analysis using a combination of CD45:FITC, cellular complexity (SSC) and LDS-751 staining. Cytogram B represents events in the nucleated cell gate (Cytogram A).

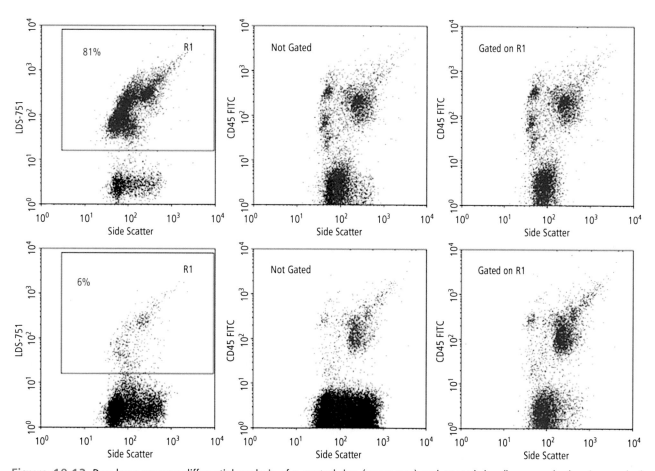

Figure 10.13 Dog bone marrow differential analysis of a control dog (upper row) and treated dog (lower row), showing marked decreases in the proportion of lymphoid and nucleated cells (R1). The latter makes the use of smears difficult: in this case collection of more events from this sample makes differential analysis possible.

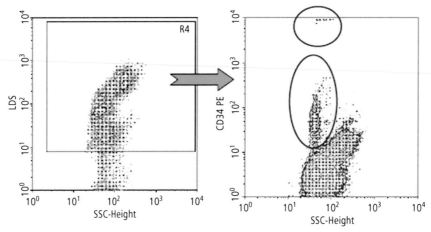

Figure 10.14 Dog bone marrow differential analysis using a combination of CD45:FITC, cellular complexity (SSC), and LDS-751 staining and CD34:PE.

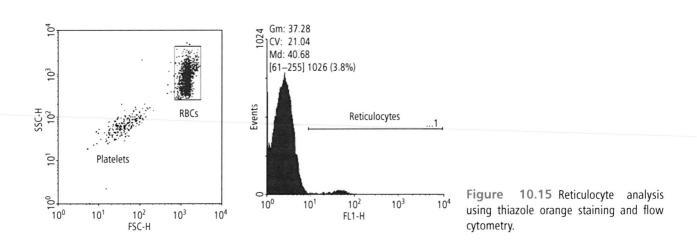

Figure 10.15 Reticulocyte analysis using thiazole orange staining and flow cytometry.

Reticulocyte analysis

Reticulocyte count in peripheral blood is a sensitive indirect indicator of bone marrow erythropoietic activity. Manual counting of reticulocytes by microscope is time consuming and associated with high degree of variation. Reticulocyte count analysis is integrated into the majority of hematology analysers. Fully automated reticulocyte analysis offers advantages relative to microscope-based scoring, including a greater number of cells analysed, much faster analysis times, less variation and a greater degree of objectivity. Reticulocytes are identified by hematology analysers using staining with methylene blue (part of Abbott and Beckman Coulter instruments), oxazine (Siemens ADVIA 120 and 2120), or fluorescent dyes such as thiazole orange (ABX), auramine O (Sysmex), CD4K530 (Abbott) or coriphosphine O (Beckman Coulter).

Assessment of neutrophil function

Flow cytometry has been employed for the assessment of various functional assays of neutrophils including oxidative burst, phagocytosis, degranulation and activation markers. Flow cytometric methods for the analysis of neutrophils and monocytes/macrophage phagocytosis and oxidative burst in different animal species have been described in several publications[6, 7, 8].

The amount of fluorescence of phagocytic cell populations was measured by flow cytometry following incubation of PMNs with fluorescent conjugated bacteria (Figure 10.16), yeasts, zymosan particles or latex beads. Assessment of oxidative burst can indirectly be evaluated by the measurement of the transformation of non-fluorescent probes (dihydrorhodamine 123) into fluorescent ones (Rhodamine 123) as a function

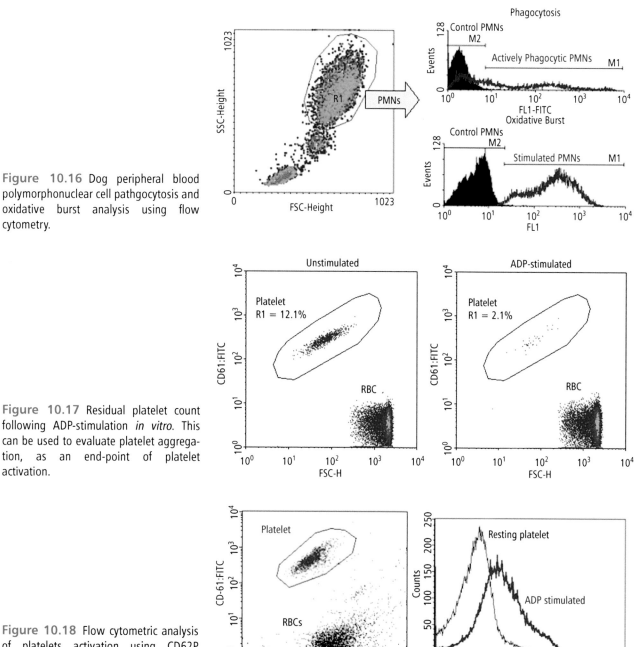

Figure 10.16 Dog peripheral blood polymorphonuclear cell pathgocytosis and oxidative burst analysis using flow cytometry.

Figure 10.17 Residual platelet count following ADP-stimulation *in vitro*. This can be used to evaluate platelet aggregation, as an end-point of platelet activation.

Figure 10.18 Flow cytometric analysis of platelets activation using CD62P (P-selectin) and CD61 (avb3, vitronectin receptor) for platelet identification.

of increased production of reactive oxygen radicals (Figure 10.16).

Platelet function assays

Some assays of platelet function are best achieved with flow cytometry, a method that allows for both enhanced analytical sensitivity and minimal mechanical manipulation during processing. Monoclonal antibodies against resting platelet surface antigens such as CD41 (gp IIb/IIIa), CD42a (gp IX), CD42b (gpIB) and CD61

are available for some animal species and can be evaluated by flow cytometry. Acquired deficiencies in these markers are associated with impaired platelet aggregation in conditions such as myelodysplasia, leukemia, aplastic anemia, marrow suppression or toxicity. Platelet activation markers, which appear on the platelet surface during activation, can also be evaluated by flow cytometry. Activation markers that are commonly used for platelet function evaluation are PAC-1, CD62P, CD 31 and CD63 (Figures 10.17 and 10.18).

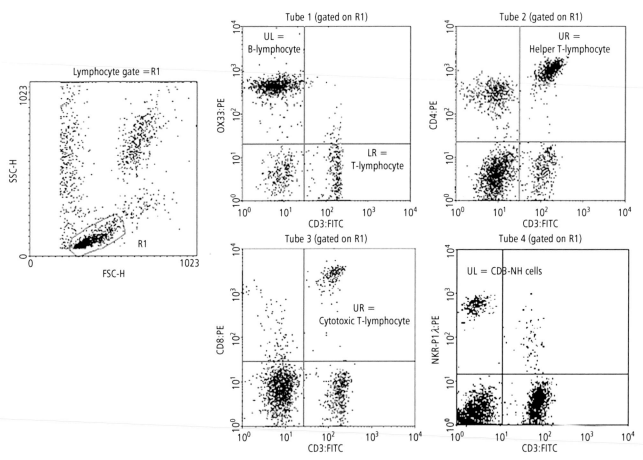

Figure 10.19 Peripheral blood lymphocyte phenotyping into B, T, T-helper, T-cytotoxic and NK lymphocytes.

Surface expression of CD62P and changes in scatter properties and platelet morphology, phosphatidylserine exposure on the platelet surface, leukocyte-platelet aggregates and microparticle formation have been used to detect activated platelets in dogs[9, 10].

Lymphocyte phenotyping

Several protocols for lymphocyte phenotyping are described in the literature for different animal species. Principally, a combination of monoclonal antibodies identifying different subpopulations of lymphocytes are added to either whole blood or lysed blood followed by washing of excess antibody and fixative. Figure 10.19 represents the flow cytometric analysis of rat lymphocytic phenotyping in whole blood.

Micronucleus

The erythrocyte micronucleus assay is a widely used regulatory assay for the assessment of chromosomal damage *in vivo*. Flow cytometric methods have been described for the scoring of micronuclei in erythro-

cytes from peripheral blood[11]. The method is based on the combination of CD71:FITC (Reticulocytes) and propidium iodide (DNA) staining. Flow cytometric scoring of micronuclei in peripheral blood reticulocytes (Figure 10.20) not only provides a rapid method with good reproducibility compared to manual scoring but also allows the integration of the micronucleus test with routine toxicological studies.

Phospholipidosis

Phospholipidosis is a phospholipid storage disorder in cells and may occur as the result of metabolic dysfunction, genetic disorder or long-term treatment with certain drugs. Potent inducers of phospholipidosis are cationic amphiphilic drugs (CAD), compounds that contain both a lipophilic moiety and ionisable nitrogen. These uncharged drugs may enter the lysosomes, become positively charged due to the acidic environment inside the lysosomes, and get trapped. Inside the lysosome the drug either forms stable complexes with phospholipids, preventing phospholipases binding

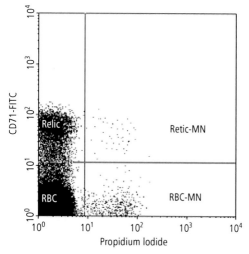

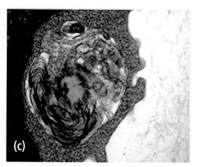

Figure 10.20 Micronucleus (MN) analysis in rat peripheral blood erythrocytes using CD71:FITC and propidium iodide staining.

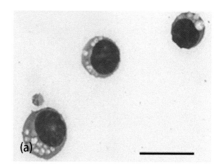

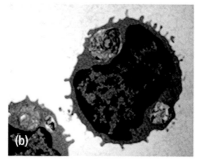

Figure 10.21 Rat peripheral blood lymphocytes exposed to cationic amphiphilic drug *in vitro* showing the presence of numerous intracytoplasmic vacuoles or myeloid bodies (EM) due to phospholipids storage disorder or phospholipidosis.

and degrading the lipids, or inhibits the phospholipases directly. The phospholipids progressively accumulate in the lysosomes; the lysosomes increase in size and contain pseudo-myelinic figures, or myeloid bodies. These figures consist of lamellar layers, which can be seen with an electron microscope (Figure 10.21).

Saad et al. (unpublished data) have utilised flow cytometry to monitor phospholipid accumulation in peripheral blood leukocytes in vitro or in vivo from several animal species. For in vivo monitoring, blood samples were taken from treated animals and the erythrocytes lysed, followed by fixation of the leukocytes. The cells were stained with Nile Red (Sigma Chemical Co., USA) and then analysed by flow cytometry to collect the forward (FSC) and side (SSC) scatter values on a linear scale and FL3 (Nile Red fluorescence) on a logarithmic scale (Figure 10.22).

Other applications

Other examples of applications of flow cytometry in comparative hematology are:

- apoptosis;
- cytotoxicity;
- cell cycle analysis;
- detection of erythrocyte-bound immunoglobulin[12];
- immunophenotyping of leukemias and lymphomas to determine cell linages and malignancy[13, 14];
- diagnosis of immune-mediated anemia and thrombocytopenia;
- detection of erythrocyte parasites[15];
- analysis of cellular composition of body cavity effusions[16];
- differential analysis of leukocytes in bovine blood and milk[17].

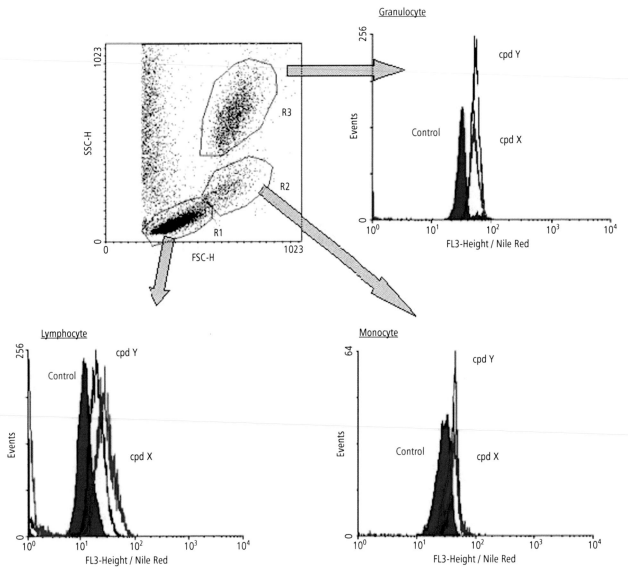

Figure 10.22 Rat peripheral blood lymphocytes exposed to cationic amphiphilic drugs in vivo and stained with Nile Red. Histogram showing shift in Nile Red fluorescence in granulocytes, monocytes and lymphocytes as compared to the histogram from control untreated animal (solid histogram).

References

1. Martin RA, Brott DA, Zandee JC, McKeel MJ (1992). Differential analysis of animal bone marrow by flow cytometry. *Cytometry* 13: 638–643.
2. Criswell KA, Bleavins MR, Zielinski D, Zandee JC (1998). Comparison of flow cytometric and manual bone marrow differentials in wistar rats. *Cytometry* 32: 9–17.
3. Saad A, Palm M, Widell S, Reiland S (2000). Differential analysis of rat bone marrow by flow cytometry. *Comp Haematol Int* 10: 97–101.
4. Schomaker SJ, Clemo FAS, Amacher DE (2002). Analysis of rat bone marrow by flow cytometry following *in vivo* exposure to cyclohexanone oxime or daunomycin HCL. *Toxicol Appl Pharmacol* 185: 48–54.
5. Weiss DJ (2004). Flow cytometric evaluation of canine bone marrow based on intracytoplasmic complexity and CD45 expression. *Vet Clin Pathol* 33(2): 96–101.
6. Saad AM and Hageltorn M (1985). Flow cytometric characterisation of bovine blood neutrophils phagocytosis of fluorescent bacteria and zymosan particles. *Acta Veterinaria Scandinavica* 26: 289–307.
7. Raidal SL, Bailey GD and Love DN (1998). The flow cytometric evaluation of phagocytosis by equine peripheral blood neutrophils and pulmonary alveolar macrophages. *Vet J* 156: 107–116.

8. Eickhoff S, Mironowa L, Carlson R, Liebold W, Tipold A (2004). Measurement of phagocytosis and oxidative burst of canine neutrophils: high variation in healthy dogs. *Veterinary Immunology and Immunopathology* 101: 109–121.

9. Wills Tb, Wardrop KJ, Meyers KM (2006). Detection of activated platelets in canine blood by use of flow cytometry. *Am J Vet Res* 67(1): 56–63.

10. Moritz A, Walcheck BK, Wiess DJ (2003). Flow cytometric detection of activated platelets in the dog. *Vet Clin Pathol* 32(1): 6–12.

11. Dertinger SD, Bishop ME, McNamee JP, Hajashi M, Suzuki T, Asano N, Nakajima M, Saito J, Moore M, Torous D, MacGregor JT (2006). Flow cytometric analysis of micronuclei in peripheral blood reticulocytes: Intra- and interlaboratory comparison with microscopic scoring. *Toxicological Sciences* 1: 83–91.

12. Kucinskiene G, Schuberth HJ, Leibold W, Pieskus J (2005). Flow cytometric evaluation of bound IgG on erythrocytes of anaemic dogs. *Vet J* 169: 303–307.

13. Weiss DJ (2001). Flow cytometric and immunophenotypic evaluation of acute lymphocytic leukemia in dog bone marrow. *J Vet Int Med* 15: 589–594.

14. Tarrant JM, Stokol T, Blue JT, McDonough SP, Farrell P (2001). Diagnosis of chronic myelogenous leukaemia in a dog using morphologic, cytochemical, and flow cytometric techniques. *Vet Clin Pathol* 30: 19–24.

15. Wyatt CR, Goff W, Davis WC (1991). A flow cytometric method for assessing viability of intraerythrocytic haemoparasites. *J Immunol Methods* 140: 23–30.

16. Moritz A, Bauer N (2005). Flow cytometric analysis of effusions in dogs and cats with the automated haematology analyser ADVIA 120. *Vet Rec* 156(21): 674–678.

17. Saad AM, Östensson K (1990). Flow cytofluorometric studies on the alteration of leukocyte populations in blood and milk during endotoxin-induced mastitis in cows. *Am J Vet Res* 51: 1603–1607.

Index

Printed and bound by CPI Group (UK) Ltd, Croydon, CR0 4YY